Richard Saitz, MD, MPH, FACP, FASAM
Marc Galanter, MD
Editors

Alcohol/Drug Screening and Brief Intervention: Advances in Evidence-Based Practice

Alcohol/Drug Screening and Brief Intervention: Advances in Evidence-Based Practice has been co-published simultaneously as *Substance Abuse*, Volume 28, Number 3 and Number 4 2007.

Pre-publication
REVIEWS,
COMMENTARIES,
EVALUATIONS . . .

"THIS IS THE RIGHT BOOK, DELIVERED AT EXACTLY THE RIGHT TIME. . . . Thought-provoking. . . . As the challenging, intelligent chapters of this book make clear, SBI is a highly promising technology, poised to enter the medical mainstream."

Eric Goplerud, PhD
Research Professor
Department of Health Policy
Director
Ensuring Solutions to Alcohol Problems
George Washington University Medical Center

Alcohol/Drug Screening and Brief Intervention: Advances in Evidence-Based Practice

Alcohol/Drug Screening and Brief Intervention: Advances in Evidence-Based Practice has been co-published simultaneously as *Substance Abuse*, Volume 28, Number 3 and Number 4 2007.

HMP

The Haworth Medical Press®
An Imprint of The Haworth Press, Inc.

www.HaworthPress.com

Monographic Separates from *Substance Abuse*™

For additional information on these and other Haworth Press titles, including descriptions, tables of contents, reviews, and prices, use the QuickSearch catalog at http://www.HaworthPress.com.

Alcohol/Drug Screening and Brief Intervention: Advances in Evidence-Based Practice, edited by Richard Saitz, MD, MPH, FACP, FASAM, and Marc Galanter, MD (Vol. 28, No. 3 and No. 4, 2007). *An examination of the latest research on substance abuse screening and brief intervention, including its effectiveness, cost-effectiveness, and methodological challenges in studying these practices.*

Alcohol/Drug Screening and Brief Intervention: Advances in Evidence-Based Practice

Richard Saitz, MD, MPH, FACP, FASAM
Marc Galanter, MD
Editors

Alcohol/Drug Screening and Brief Intervention: Advances in Evidence-Based Practice has been co-published simultaneously as *Substance Abuse*, Volume 28, Number 3 and Number 4 2007.

HMP

The Haworth Medical Press®
An Imprint of The Haworth Press, Inc.

www.HaworthPress.com

Published by

The Haworth Medical Press®, 10 Alice Street, Binghamton, NY 13904-1580 USA

The Haworth Medical Press® is an imprint of The Haworth Press, Inc., 10 Alice Street, Binghamton, NY 13904-1580 USA.

Alcohol/Drug Screening and Brief Intervention: Advances in Evidence-Based Practice has been co-published simultaneously as *Substance Abuse*, Volume 28, Number 3 and Number 4 2007.

Library of Congress Cataloging-in-Publication Data

Alcohol/drug screening and brief intervention : advances in evidence-based practice / Richard Saitz, Marc Galanter, editors.
p. ; cm.
"Co-published simultaneously as Substance abuse, volume 28, number 3 and number 4 2007."
Includes bibliographical references and index.
ISBN 978-0-7890-3749-7 (soft cover : alk. paper)
1. Alcoholism–United States. 2. Substance abuse–United States. 3. Medical screening–United States. 4. Brief psychotherapy–United States. 5. Evidence-based psychiatry–United States. I. Saitz, Richard. II. Galanter, Marc. III. Substanve abuse.
[DNLM: 1. Substance-Related Disorders–diagnosis. 2. Counseling. 3. Evidence-Based Medicine. 4. Mass Screening. 5. Psychotherapy, Brief. 6. Substance-Related Disorders–therapy. W1 SU147G v.28 no.3-4 2007 / WM 270 A3562 2007]
RC565.7.A52 2007
362.292′0973–dc22

2007042198

The HAWORTH PRESS *Inc*

Abstracting, Indexing & Outward Linking

PRINT *and* ELECTRONIC BOOKS & JOURNALS

This section provides you with a list of major indexing & abstracting services and other tools for bibliographic access. That is to say, each service began covering this periodical during the year noted in the right column. Most Websites which are listed below have indicated that they will either post, disseminate, compile, archive, cite, or alert their own Website users with research-based content from this work. (This list is as current as the copyright date of this publication.)

Abstracting, Website/Indexing Coverage . . . . Year When Coverage Began

- ***International Bibliography of Book Reviews on the Humanities and Social Sciences (IBR) (Thomson) <http://www.saur.de>*** **2006**
- ***(CAB ABSTRACTS, CABI) <http://www.cabi.org>*** **2004**
- *****Academic Search Premier (EBSCO)** <http://search.ebscohost.com>*** **2007**
- *****CINAHL (Cumulative Index to Nursing & Allied Health Literature) (EBSCO)** <http://www.cinahl.com>*** **1995**
- *****CINAHL Plus (EBSCO)** <http://search.ebscohost.com>*** **2007**
- *****Educational Research Abstracts (ERA) (Taylor & Francis)** <http://www.tandf.co.uk/era>*** **2007**
- *****EMBASE Excerpta Medica (Elsevier)** <http://www.elsevier.nl>*** **2003**
- *****EMBASE.com (The Power of EMBASE + MEDLINE Combined) (Elsevier)** <http://www.embase.com>*** **2003**
- *****MEDLINE (National Library of Medicine)** <http://www.nlm.nih.gov>*** **2002**
- *****Psychological Abstracts (PsycINFO)** <http://www.apa.org>*** **1995**
- *****PubMed** <http://www.ncbi.nlm.nih.gov/pubmed/>*** **2002**
- *****Social Work Abstracts (NASW)** <http://www.silverplatter.com/catalog/swab.htm>*** **1997**
- ***Abstracts in Anthropology <http://www.baywood.com/Journals/PreviewJournals.asp?Id=0001-3455>*** **2006**
- ***Abstracts on Hygiene and Communicable Diseases (CAB ABSTRACTS, CABI) <http://www.cabi.org>*** **2006**
- ***Academic Search Alumni Edition (EBSCO) <http://search.ebscohost.com>*** **2007**
- ***Academic Search Complete (EBSCO) <http://search.ebscohost.com>*** **2007**
- ***Academic Source Premier (EBSCO) <http://search.ebscohost.com>*** **2007**
- ***Addiction Abstracts (Published in collaboration with the National Addiction Centre & Carfax, Taylor & Francis) <http://www.tandf.co.uk/addiction-abs>*** **2007**
- ***Alcohol Studies Database <http://cf7-test.scc-net.rutgers.edu/alcohol_studies/alcohol/index.htm>*** **2007**

(continued)

- *AMED Database (Allied & Complementary Medicine Database)* **2004**
- *British Library Inside (The British Library) <http://www.bl.uk/services/current/inside.html>* **2006**
- *Child Development Abstractrs (Taylor & Francis) <http://www.tandf.co.uk/>* **2007**
- *Contents Pages in Education (Taylor & Francis) <http://www.tandf.co.uk>* **2007**
- *DH-Data (available via DataStar and in the HMIC [Health Management Information Consortium] CD ROM) <http://www.dh.gov.uk/Home/fs/en>* **2005**
- *DrugScope <http://www.drugscope.org.uk/resources/researchaids/journals.htm>* **2007**
- *EBSCOhost Electronic Journals Service (EJS) <http://search.ebscohost.com>* **2004**
- *Educational Management Abstracts (Taylor & Francis) <http://www.tandf.co.uk>* **2007**
- *Educational Technology Abstracts (Taylor & Francis) <http://www.tandf.co.uk>* **2007**
- *Electronic Collections Online (OCLC) <http://www.oclc.org/electroniccollections/>* **2006**
- *Elsevier Eflow-I* **2006**
- *Elsevier Scopus <http://www.info.scopus.com>* **2005**
- *EMCare (Elsevier) <http://www.elsevier.com>* **2006**
- *Family Index Database <http://www.familyscholar.com>* **2004**
- *Family Violence & Sexual Assault Bulletin* **2006**
- *Google <http://www.google.com>* **2004**
- *Google Scholar <http://scholar.google.com>* **2004**
- *Haworth Document Delivery Center <http://www.HaworthPress.com/journals/dds.asp>* **2004**
- *HealthSTAR (Ovid)* **2006**
- *Human Resources Abstracts (Sage)* **2004**
- *IndexCopernicus <http://www.indexcopernicus.com>* **2006**
- *International Bibliography of Periodical Literature on the Humanities and Social Sciences (IBZ) (Thomson) <http://www.saur.de>* **2006**
- *JournalSeek <http://www.journalseek.net>* **2006**
- *Links@Ovid (via CrossRef targeted DOI links) <http://www.ovid.com>* **2005**
- *Medical Benefits <http://www.aspenpublishers.com>* **2007**
- *Multicultural Education Abstracts (Taylor & Francis) <http://www.tandf.co.uk>* **2007**
- *NewJour (Electronic Journals & Newsletters) <http://gort.ucsd.edu/newjour/>* **2006**
- *OCLC ArticleFirst <http://www.oclc.org/services/databases/>* **2006**
- *Ovid Linksolver (OpenURL link resolver via CrossRef targeted DOI links) <http://www.linksolver.com>* **2005**
- *Project MAINSTREAM <http://www.projectmainstream.net>* **2005**
- *PubsHub.com > (Outward Linking) <http://www.PubsHub.com>* **2007**
- *Referativnyi Zhurnal (Abstracts Journal of the All-Russian Institute of Scientific and Technical Information-in Russian) <http://www.viniti.ru>* **2006**
- *Research into Higher Education Abstracts (Taylor & Francis) <http://www.tandf.co.uk>* . . . **2007**
- *SafetyLit <http://www.safetylit.org>* **2004**
- *Sage Family Studies Abstracts* **2004**

(continued)

- *SALIS (Substance Abuse Librarians & Information Specialists) Alcohol, Tobacco & Other Drug Journals on the Web <http://www.salis.org/resources/atod_journals.html>* **2007**
- *Scopus (See instead Elsevier Scopus) <http://www.info.scopus.com>* **2005**
- *Sociedad Iberoamericana de Información Científica (SIIC) <http://www.siicsalud.com/>* . . . **2006**
- *SocIndex (EBSCO) <http://search.ebscohost.com>* **2007**
- *SocINDEX with Full Text (EBSCO) <http://search.ebscohost.com>* **2007**
- *Sociology of Education Abstracst (Taylor & Francis) <http://www.tandf.co.uk>* **2007**
- *Special Educational Needs Abstracts (Taylor & Francis) <http://www.tandf.co.uk>* **2007**
- *Studies on Women and Gender Abstracts (Taylor & Francis) <http://www.tandf.co.uk/swa>* **2006**
- *SwetsWise <http://www.swets.com>* **2005**
- *Technical Education & Training Abstracts (Taylor & Francis) <http://www.tandf.co.uk>* . . . **2007**
- *Tropical Diseases Bulletin (CAB ABSTRACTS, CABI) <http://www.cabi.org>* **2006**
- *Violence and Abuse Abstracts (Sage)* **1997**
- *zetoc (The British Library) <http://www.bl.uk>* **2004**

Bibliographic Access

- *ATForum.com <http://www.atforum.com>*
- *Cabell's Directory of Publishing Opportunities in Psychology <http://www.cabells.com>*
- *MediaFinder <http://www.mediafinder.com/>*
- *Ulrich's Periodicals Directory: The Global Source for Periodicals Information Since 1932 <http://www.bowkerlink.com>*

Special Bibliographic Notes related to special journal issues (separates) and indexing/abstracting:

- indexing/abstracting services in this list will also cover material in any "separate" that is co-published simultaneously with Haworth's special thematic journal issue or DocuSerial. Indexing/abstracting usually covers material at the article/chapter level.
- monographic co-editions are intended for either non-subscribers or libraries which intend to purchase a second copy for their circulating collections.
- monographic co-editions are reported to all jobbers/wholesalers/approval plans. The source journal is listed as the "series" to assist the prevention of duplicate purchasing in the same manner utilized for books-in-series.
- to facilitate user/access services all indexing/abstracting services are encouraged to utilize the co-indexing entry note indicated at the bottom of the first page of each article/chapter/contribution.
- this is intended to assist a library user of any reference tool (whether print, electronic, online, or CD-ROM) to locate the monographic version if the library has purchased this version but not a subscription to the source journal.
- individual articles/chapters in any Haworth publication are also available through the Haworth Document Delivery Service (HDDS).

As part of Haworth's continuing commitment to better serve our library patrons, we are proud to be working with the following electronic services:

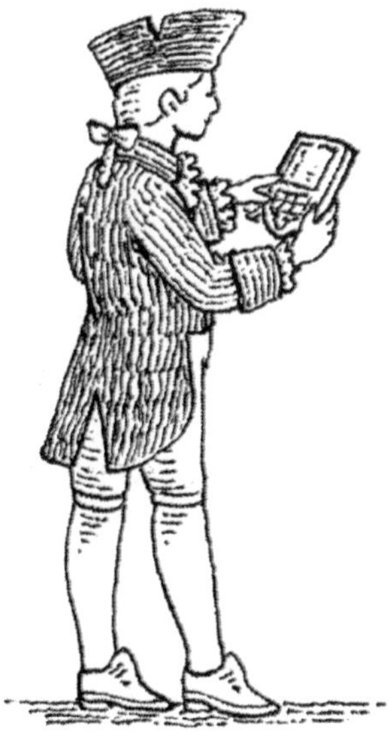

AGGREGATOR SERVICES

- EBSCOhost
- Ingenta
- J-Gate
- Minerva
- OCLC FirstSearch
- Oxmill
- SwetsWise

LINK RESOLVER SERVICES

- 1Cate (Openly Informatics)
- ChemPort (American Chemical Society)
- CrossRef
- Gold Rush (Coalliance)
- LinkOut (PubMed)
- LINKplus (Atypon)
- LinkSolver (Ovid)
- LinkSource with A-to-Z (EBSCO)
- Resource Linker (Ulrich)
- SerialsSolutions (ProQuest)
- SFX (Ex Libris)
- Sirsi Resolver (SirsiDynix)
- Tour (TDnet)
- Vlink (Extensity, formerly Geac)
- WebBridge (Innovative Interfaces)

Alcohol/Drug Screening and Brief Intervention: Advances in Evidence-Based Practice

CONTENTS

EXAMPLES OF WHERE IT HAS BEEN APPLIED

ABOUT THE EDITORS

Richard Saitz, MD, MPH, is a primary care general internist and health services researcher. He is Professor of Medicine and Epidemiology, Boston University Schools of Medicine and Public Health, and Director of the Clinical Addiction Research and Education Unit of the Section of General Internal Medicine at Boston Medical Center. He is a Fellow of both the American College of Physicians and the American Society of Addiction Medicine. He is also Associate Director of the National Institute on Alcohol Abuse and Alcoholism's Youth Alcohol Prevention Center. His research–supported by the National Institutes of Health (NIH)–focuses on unhealthy alcohol use in people in general health settings. Areas of particular emphasis are: Screening and brief counseling for unhealthy alcohol use in primary care settings, quality of care related to unhealthy alcohol use, motivational interviewing for health behavior change, web-based interventions, and addiction disease management/integrating substance dependence treatment and primary medical care. He is President of the Association for Medical Education and Research in Substance Abuse (AMERSA), a national interdisciplinary organization of health professions faculty educators and researchers. He is also Associate Director of the Boston University Medical Center's Office of Clinical Research.

Dr. Saitz has been Chairman of the Institutional Review Board at Boston University, and was selected as one of Ten Outstanding Young Leaders by the Boston Jaycees in 2003. He has been a member of the Steering Committee of the international Motivational Interviewing Network of Trainers. His research has included randomized clinical trials, survey research, large database studies, and prospective cohort studies, with NIH, other federal and foundation support for his work (the latter as a Generalist Physician Faculty Scholar). He has mentored numerous research trainees and has led a number of educational efforts including clinical research training, and alcohol science education projects.

Marc Galanter, MD, is Professor of Psychiatry at NYU, Founding Director of the Division of Alcoholism and Drug Abuse at NYU and Bellevue Hospital, and Director of the NYU Fellowship Training Program in Addiction Psychiatry. He is also Division Director at NYU's World Health Organization Collaborating Center, and Director of its national Center for Medical Fellowships in Alcoholism and Drug Abuse. In addition to 267 articles, chapters, and books, he is Editor of the "Textbook of Substance Abuse Treatment."

He attended Albert Einstein College of Medicine where he did his residency in psychiatry. After that he was Clinical Associate at the National Institute of Mental Health, and then an NIH Career Teacher. He later served as President of the Association for Medical Education and Research in Substance Abuse (AMERSA) (1976-7), the American Academy of Addiction Psychiatry (1991-2), and the American Society of Addiction Medicine (1999-2001).

Dr. Galanter's research and teaching interests have focused on addiction treatment, spirituality, and improving treatment systems. His current NIH and foundation-funded studies address family therapy for substance abuse, pharmacologic treatment for narcotic addiction, and self-help modalities. His Center at NYU has prepared curricula for 46 teaching hospitals and affiliated medical schools.

Among his awards are the Gold Achievement Award for innovation in clinical care and the Seymour Vestermark Award for Psychiatric Education, both from the American Psychiatric Association, and the McGovern Award for medical teaching from AMERSA.

ALL HAWORTH MEDICAL PRESS BOOKS
AND JOURNALS ARE PRINTED
ON CERTIFIED ACID-FREE PAPER

Introduction: Screening and Brief Intervention

Richard Saitz, MD, MPH

Any approach to addressing unhealthy alcohol and drug use that does not include attention beyond those with substance dependence who receive specialty treatment misses the majority of people affected. More people use substances and risk future consequences, or use them and have had consequences that do not meet the threshold of a disorder, than meet criteria for the substance use disorders abuse and dependence. Most people with dependence do not seek or receive specialty treatment or 12-step help. And mutual help approaches and most specialty treatments are not applicable to those without dependence.

Screening and brief intervention can have a major role in reducing risk for those with nondependent unhealthy use and referring those who need it to specialty treatment. Screening tests have been developed and validated to identify the spectrum of unhealthy use. These tests do not diagnose disease; rather they identify people with a high likelihood of having a substance-related condition. Early tests such as the CAGE alcohol-screening questionnaire were validated to identify people with alcohol dependence. More recently, researchers have recognized the need to identify the whole spectrum of unhealthy use and have validated questionnaires for that purpose, such as single-item screening questions or longer questionnaires such as the Alcohol Use Disorders Identification Test (AUDIT). These tools identify people with a wide range of severity who then require an assessment to determine next steps. The assessment should address not only the presence or absence of dependence, but also the level of readiness to change or seek further help. This latter assessment is critical in those identified by screening, in contrast to those who present for care having recognized a problem and who have decided to seek help. A brief counseling intervention can, in the case of those with nondependent unhealthy alcohol use, decrease alcohol use and even related problems. For those not ready to change, the goal is to increase motivation. For those with dependence, the goal is referral to additional help when the patient is ready. For those seeking treatment, brief intervention has not been shown to be inferior to longer durations of care.

What is a brief intervention? A brief intervention is counseling that takes about 10 to 15 minutes, usually on a few occasions (though some have included sessions up to 30-60 minutes repeated 4 or more times). The counseling includes feedback about personal risk, emphasis on the patient's responsibility for change, explicit advice to change, provision of a variety of ways to change (a menu of options), an empathic style, and support of a patient's perception of self-efficacy or optimism that they can change.

Richard Saitz is affiliated with Section of General Internal Medicine, Boston Medical Center, 91 East Concord Street, Suit #200, Boston, MA 02118-2644 (E-mail: rsaitz@bu.edu).

[Haworth co-indexing entry note]: "Introduction: Screening and Brief Intervention." Saitz, Richard. Co-published simultaneously in *Substance Abuse* (The Haworth Medical Press, an imprint of The Haworth Press, Inc.) Vol. 28, No. 3, 2007, pp. 1-2; and: *Alcohol/Drug Screening and Brief Intervention: Advances in Evidence-Based Practice* (ed: Richard Saitz, and Marc Galanter) The Haworth Medical Press, an imprint of The Haworth Press, Inc., 2007, pp. 1-2. Single or multiple copies of this article are available for a fee from The Haworth Document Delivery Service [1-800-HAWORTH, 9:00 a.m. - 5:00 p.m. (EST). E-mail address: docdelivery@haworthpress.com].

Available online at http://suba.haworthpress.com

doi:10.1300/J465v28n03_01

Screening and brief intervention have great promise. The skills can be learned and delivered by health professionals in many disciplines. Unlike more intensive treatments, these approaches can be implemented in general health care settings. Screening and brief intervention can identify and intervene with people who have not sought care for their substance use, and therefore might prevent progression from risky use to use with consequences or dependence.

The efficacy of screening and brief intervention has been best demonstrated in adults with nondependent unhealthy alcohol use in primary medical care settings. Study results are less clear in other settings and for other substances. In this special publication of *Substance Abuse*, articles review the literature on screening and brief intervention, effectiveness and cost-effectiveness and methodological challenges in studying these practices. The articles also report on how to measure the use of screening and brief intervention in practice, the multiple risk factor context in which unhealthy alcohol use occurs, clinician training, the best ways to screen adolescents, and which patients are most likely to change. Finally, a paper reviews what we know about a way to expand screening and brief intervention beyond the office–by delivering services via the web. Screening and brief intervention are being implemented in many settings now–hospitals, primary care settings, trauma centers, college health services and beyond. They have been around for more than 40 years and are recognized practices. As such, they require critical re-evaluation as they become more widely disseminated. This special issue addresses both background and future challenges for screening and brief intervention for unhealthy substance use.

OVERVIEW

Screening and Brief Intervention Enter Their 5th Decade

Richard Saitz, MD, MPH

SUMMARY. About 40 years since the first controlled study, screening and brief intervention (SBI) are being disseminated into practice. But many unanswered questions remain. Studies in this special issue address what we know and don't know about alcohol and drug SBI, cost-effectiveness, patient preferences, education for clinicians, quality performance measures, "no-contact" SBI, predictors of behavior change, and methodological concerns with the SBI literature. The best evidence for efficacy of SBI is that it can lead to decreased consumption in primary care patients with non-dependent unhealthy alcohol use. But further research is needed on brief drug screening tools, efficacy of SBI for drugs, effectiveness in real world settings, integration of SBI for alcohol and drugs with other health behaviors, effects of SBI on alcohol and drug consequences, effects on dependence among those not seeking help, and on how to best disseminate the efficacious elements of SBI into practice. doi:10.1300/J465v28n03_02 *[Article copies available for a fee from The Haworth Document Delivery Service: 1-800-HAWORTH. E-mail address: <docdelivery@haworthpress.com> Website: <http://www.HaworthPress.com> © 2007 by The Haworth Press, Inc. All rights reserved.]*

KEYWORDS. Screening and brief intervention (SBI), patient preference, alcohol use, drug use, behavior change

Given meta-analyses demonstrating efficacy (1,2), a "B" recommendation from the US Preventive Services Task Force (USPSTF) (3), large US Federal demonstration programs (4),

Richard Saitz is affiliated with the Clinical Addiction Research and Education (CARE) Unit, Section of General Internal Medicine, Boston Medical Center and Boston University School of Medicine, Boston, MA and the Youth Alcohol Prevention Center, Department of Epidemiology, Boston University School of Public Health, Boston, MA.

Address correspondence to: Richard Saitz, MD, MPH, Boston Medical Center, 91 East Concord Street, Suite #200, Boston, MA 02118 (E-mail: rsaitz@bu.edu).

Support from the National Institute on Alcohol Abuse and Alcoholism (R-01s AA 10870 12617, 13304, 14713, 14258, R25 AA 13822, and P60 AA 13759), the National Institute on Drug Abuse (R-01 DA 10019 and R25 13582), the National Center for Research Resources (K30 22252), and the Substance Abuse and Mental Health Services Administration (U79TI018311).

[Haworth co-indexing entry note]: "Screening and Brief Intervention Enter Their 5th Decade." Saitz, Richard. Co-published simultaneously in *Substance Abuse* (The Haworth Medical Press, an imprint of The Haworth Press, Inc.) Vol. 28, No. 3, 2007, pp. 3-6; and: *Alcohol/Drug Screening and Brief Intervention: Advances in Evidence-Based Practice* (ed: Richard Saitz, and Marc Galanter) The Haworth Medical Press, an imprint of The Haworth Press, Inc., 2007, pp. 3-6. Single or multiple copies of this article are available for a fee from The Haworth Document Delivery Service [1-800-HAWORTH, 9:00 a.m. - 5:00 p.m. (EST). E-mail address: docdelivery@haworthpress.com].

Available online at http://suba.haworthpress.com

doi:10.1300/J465v28n03_02

and new billing codes from the US Center for Medicare and Medicaid Services (CMS) (5), one might think that there are few unanswered questions about screening and brief intervention (SBI) for unhealthy substance use, particularly about efficacy. Now in its fifth decade (if one dates its birth from a controlled trial in people with alcoholism in an emergency department who were not seeking alcohol treatment) (6), SBI has been studied extensively and is on the verge of widespread dissemination. Of note, although the call for this issue was not specific to alcohol, most of the authors responded with alcohol-focused papers, consistent with the published research.

One of the first studies of SBI appeared in 1961 (6). Chafetz reported that people with alcoholism were more likely to follow-up in an alcohol clinic after brief advice from a psychiatrist in an emergency department, than after no advice. These results were promising because they suggested that a brief intervention could have some impact on people with a complex chronic disease. But this early study generated many questions, some of which have been answered by dozens of clinical trials and other studies over the past 30-40 years. In this special issue, a wide range of papers cover what we know and what we don't know about screening and brief intervention, and point the way towards cutting edge research and thoughtful practice and policy in this area.

Babor and colleagues in a comprehensive review, detail evidence for the validity of screening tests and for the efficacy of brief intervention. In so doing they expand the discussion to include "brief treatments." They find that evidence is available supporting the validity of alcohol screening questionnaires but the review does not identify brief valid drug screening tests for use in general healthcare settings. They also find evidence lacking in the areas of brief intervention for drug use and disorders, brief interventions whose goal is to link people with dependence to specialized treatment, and on how to disseminate known effective approaches widely. Several other papers in this issue begin to address some of these gaps.

Most of the papers in this publication are relevant to implementation and more widespread dissemination of SBI. For example, Kraemer, in reviewing the costs and outcomes associated with SBI, finds that much of the literature indicates favorable cost-benefit comparisons, at least for unhealthy alcohol use. But he also points the way forward, encouraging the development of analyses that will allow SBI to be compared with other health interventions. Funderburk et al. point out that few studies of alcohol brief intervention have considered or included attention to other risk factors for health consequences. Yet most patients in primary care settings have multiple risk factors and unhealthy alcohol use is among the most common of these risk factors. Their findings suggest a need to study alcohol SBI in the context of other common health problems and to address issues of efficacy and prioritization. Knight et al. also addressed a practical issue in their study of screening adolescents for substance use. It appears that adolescents prefer screening by written questionnaire to screening by a nurse or doctor. If they were to be screened by a clinician, however, they would prefer one that they know. For a universal practice (SBI), these data are quite useful for planning.

The Academic ED SBIRT Research Collaborative, as part of efforts to implement SBI in selected emergency departments nationally, tested a relatively brief educational program finding that practitioners who experienced it were more likely to report using SBI. Although the study design and small absolute impact of the education program limit the conclusions that can be drawn, their report suggests that widely disseminated SBI education is feasible, but that large changes in practice will require changes in infrastructure.

Bradley et al. are looking to the future, in which alcohol screening and brief intervention are measured as markers of quality care. They and their colleagues (Hawkins et al.) point out the strengths and limitations of various data sources for measuring performance. In doing so, they are forced to do something the literature has done inconsistently to date–they define the features that must be present in order to call an interaction a brief intervention: feedback and advice. Their work also suggests that methods for determining who has unhealthy alcohol use and whether they receive brief intervention are not only for focused scientists. The differences in detection between systematic survey and clinical documentation even in a system with a high penetration of screening are big enough to create problems if they are ignored in quality of care and performance measurement.

But methodologic concerns like those should be of great interest to SBI researchers, clinicians and policymakers. Kypri points out common limitations in published SBI research and suggests ways to improve designs for future trials. Among many recommendations, he reminds us that within group comparisons should never be used to prove efficacy, since improvements can be related to natural history in people who have agreed to enter a study of behavior change. Addressing the limitations he has delineated is critical so that we can clarify the true magnitude, benefits and risks of SBI.

Finally, Zisserson et al. review a strategy through which SBI could reach a broader audience. They systematically reviewed studies of brief intervention without direct real time contact with an interventionist, primarily studies of web-based brief intervention for college students. With effect sizes as large or larger than in-person interventions, the provocative question arises as to whether these approaches should be covered by health insurers. As with many reviews, however, they raise almost as many questions as they answer. Although the results of the studies are promising (in favor of web-based SBI efficacy) they also noted that studies were small, few in number, and inconsistent. These findings indicate a need for more definitive efficacy studies, and the need to understand the ideal duration and frequency of these interventions, and their necessary components. To that end, Daeppen and colleagues have discovered one characteristic of brief intervention that is predictive of later success. And it is not a characteristic of the intervention or the interventionist; rather, it appears to be the patient's intention to change, consistent with other recent observational data (7).

US Federal programs report significant declines in substance use after screening almost half a million Americans in general healthcare settings (8). Of at-risk, high-risk, or severe-risk individuals, 62 percent reported stopping drug use and 60 percent reduced their alcohol consumption to low-risk levels (4). But these observational data, while dramatic and hopeful, cannot reflect the true efficacy of SBI. The best evidence for SBI is for decreases in consumption (not consequences) by people reporting non-dependent unhealthy alcohol use. In these patients, meta-analysis finds 12% declines in unhealthy use (2), and decreases in use of about 5 grams per day (1), in primary care settings. How these decreases translate into important clinical outcomes has been studied little, though some reports suggest recurrent trauma, motor vehicle crashes, and even mortality might be decreased (9-11). But in some settings (e.g., emergency departments and general hospitals) there is growing evidence that SBI for alcohol does not have efficacy (12,13). For non-dependent unhealthy alcohol use we need studies that identify more potent interventions and that find ways to disseminate SBI into practice.

But what about SBI for other drugs? Important drivers of practice in this area do not recommend universal SBI. For example, the National Quality Forum recommends alcohol but not drug screening (14). Based on published controlled studies, the USPSTF recommends screening and brief intervention not for drugs, but for alcohol misuse (by which they mean, unlike Bradley et al.'s use of the term to mean the spectrum including dependence, nondependent unhealthy use) (3). A USPSTF update on drug screening is in progress (15). Only one large randomized trial supports drug SBI, finding a 4% increase in cocaine or heroin abstinence (16). The demand for controlled studies in this area (as in other areas of health) is not simply an academic concern–there are reasons why drug SBI may not live up to its promise, and why alcohol SBI study results may not apply to other drugs. Although substances of abuse may have much in common, screening for one substance versus a list of varied drugs presents a challenge. Unlike for alcohol, there is no very brief (e.g., 1-4 items) drug-screening questionnaire that has been well validated for use in general healthcare settings. The severity of addiction in drug users identified by screening may be higher than among screening-identified unhealthy users of alcohol, and may vary by substance (e.g., marijuana, opioids, methamphetamine) (16). As a result SBI may have less impact on drug compared to alcohol use. Methodological issues may also be even more of a challenge for drug SBI studies since self-report of drug use has different implications than report of alcohol use. Finally, while the outcome of less drinking has been achieved with alcohol SBI, the clinical value of "less drug use" is uncertain.

Because SBI has reached middle age, and because of the potential for widespread dissemination into practice, we must pause and critically consider the scientific evidence. Articles in this issue are a solid start for this process. Universal alcohol SBI is mature. As a result, we need studies of dissemination (including large simple pragmatic or effectiveness trials, and systems interventions), integration with other health behavior interventions, and studies of those with dependence who are not seeking treatment. To get to the same point with drug SBI we need validation studies of screening tests in general healthcare settings, and controlled clinical trials that test efficacy so we can avoid wasted efforts and even harm. A failure to thoughtfully review where we are, risks overzealous dissemination, and threatens opportunities to expand proven substance-related services throughout the health system.

REFERENCES

1. Bertholet N, Daeppen JB, Wietlisbach V, Fleming M, Burnand B. Reduction of alcohol consumption by brief alcohol intervention in primary care: systematic review and meta-analysis. Arch Intern Med 2005; 165:986-995.

2. Beich A, Thorsen T, Rollnick S. Screening in brief intervention trials targeting excessive drinkers in general practice: systematic review and meta-analysis. BMJ 2003;327:536-542.

3. US Preventive Services Task Force. Screening and behavioral counseling interventions in primary care to reduce alcohol misuse: recommendation statement. Ann Intern Med. 2004;140:554-56.

4. Substance Abuse and Mental Health Services Administration (SAMHSA) News. Screening adds prevention to treatment. January/February 2006;14(1):1. http://www.samhsa.gov/SAMHSA_NEWS/VolumeXIV_1/index.htm accessed January 20, 2007.

5. Medicare Learning Matters (MLN). http://www.cms.hhs.gov/MLNMattersArticles/downloads/MM5255.pdf accessed January 20, 2007.

6. Chafetz ME. A procedure for establishing therapeutic contact with the alcoholic. Q J Stud Alcohol 1961;22:325-328.

7. Amrhein PC, Miller WR, Yahne CE, Palmer M, Fulcher L. Client commitment language during motivational interviewing predicts drug use outcomes. J Consult Clin Psychol 2003;71:862-878.

8. ONDCP and ACCME collaborate on screening and brief intervention as model for continuing medical education (press release). http://www.whitehousedrugpolicy.gov/news/press07/011207.html accessed January 20, 2007.

9. Gentilello LM, Rivara FP, Donovan DM, Jurkovich GJ, Daranciang E, Dunn CW, Villaveces A, Copass M, Ries RR. Alcohol interventions in a trauma center as a means of reducing the risk of injury recurrence. Ann Surg 1999;230:473-480.

10. Fleming MF, Mundt MP, French MT, Manwell LB, Stauffacher EA, Barry KL. Brief physician advice for problem drinkers: longterm efficacy and benefit-cost analysis. Alcohol Clin Exp Res 2002;26:36-43.

11. Kristenson H, Osterling A, Nilsson JA, Lindgarde F. Prevention of alcohol-related deaths in middle-aged heavy drinkers. Alcohol Clin Exp Res 2002;26:478-484.

12. D'Onofrio G, Degutis LC, Fiellin DA, Pantalon MV, Busch SH, Chawarski MC, O'Connor PG. Emergency practitioner performed brief intervention for harmful and hazardous drinkers in the emergency department. Alcohol Clin Exp Res 2005;29(suppl): 179A.

13. Saitz R, Palfai TP, Cheng DM, Horton NJ, Freedner N, Dukes K, Kraemer KL, Roberts MS, Guerriero RT, Samet JH. Brief intervention for medical inpatients with unhealthy alcohol use: a randomized controlled trial. Ann Intern Med 2007;146(3):167-176.

14. Power EJ, Nishimi RY, Kizer KW. Evidence-based treatment practices for substance use disorders. National Quality Forum. Washington DC: 2005.

15. U.S. Preventive Services Task Force, Screening for Drug Abuse. http://www.ahrq.gov/clinic/uspstf/uspsdrug.htm accessed January 20, 2007.

16. Bernstein J, Bernstein E, Tassiopoulos K, Heeren T, Levenson S, Hingson R. Brief motivational intervention at a clinic visit reduces cocaine and heroin use. Drug Alcohol Depend 2005;77:49-59.

doi:10.1300/J465v28n03_02

Screening, Brief Intervention, and Referral to Treatment (SBIRT): Toward a Public Health Approach to the Management of Substance Abuse

Thomas F. Babor, PhD, MPH
Bonnie G. McRee, MPH
Patricia A. Kassebaum, MA
Paul L. Grimaldi, PhD
Kazi Ahmed, PhD
Jeremy Bray, PhD

SUMMARY. Screening, Brief Intervention, and Referral to Treatment (SBIRT) is a comprehensive and integrated approach to the delivery of early intervention and treatment services through universal screening for persons with substance use disorders and those at risk. This paper describes research on the components of SBIRT conducted during the past 25 years, including the development of screening tests, clinical trials of brief interventions and implementation research. Beginning in the 1980s, concerted efforts were made in the US and at the World Health Organization to provide an evidence base for alcohol screening and brief intervention in primary health care settings. With the development of reliable and accurate screening tests for alcohol, more than a hundred clinical trials were conducted to evaluate the efficacy and cost effectiveness of alcohol screening and brief intervention in primary care, emergency departments and trauma centers. With the accumulation of positive evidence, implementation research on alcohol SBI was begun in the 1990s, followed by trials of similar methods for other substances (e.g., illicit drugs, tobacco, prescription drugs) and by national demonstration programs in the US and other countries. The results of these efforts demonstrate the cumulative benefit of translational research on health care delivery systems and substance abuse policy. That SBIRT yields short-term improvements in individuals' health is irrefutable; long-term effects on population health have not yet been demonstrated, but simulation models suggest that the benefits could be substantial. doi:10.1300/J465v28n03_03 *[Article copies available for a fee from The Haworth Document Delivery Service: 1-800-HAWORTH. E-mail address: <docdelivery@haworthpress.com> Website: <http://www.HaworthPress.com> © 2007 by The Haworth Press, Inc. All rights reserved.]*

Thomas F. Babor and Bonnie G. McRee are affiliated with the University of Connecticut School of Medicine.

Patricia A. Kassebaum, Paul L. Grimaldi, and Kazi Ahmed are affiliated with JBS International, Inc., Silver Spring, MD.

Jeremy Bray is affiliated with RTI International, Research Triangle Park, NC.

Address correspondence to: Thomas F. Babor, The University of Connecticut School of Medicine, 263 Farmington Avenue, Farmington, CT 06030 (E-mail: babor@nso.uchc.edu).

The writing of this paper was supported by the Center for Substance Abuse Treatment, Substance Abuse and Mental Health Services Administration [SBIRT Contract No. is 270-03-1000 and the Task Order No. is 270-03-1007].

[Haworth co-indexing entry note]: "Screening, Brief Intervention, and Referral to Treatment (SBIRT): Toward a Public Health Approach to the Management of Substance Abuse." Babor, Thomas F. et al. Co-published simultaneously in *Substance Abuse* (The Haworth Medical Press, an imprint of The Haworth Press, Inc.) Vol. 28, No. 3, 2007, pp. 7-30; and: *Alcohol/Drug Screening and Brief Intervention: Advances in Evidence-Based Practice* (ed: Richard Saitz, and Marc Galanter) The Haworth Medical Press, an imprint of The Haworth Press, Inc., 2007, pp. 7-30. Single or multiple copies of this article are available for a fee from The Haworth Document Delivery Service [1-800-HAWORTH, 9:00 a.m. - 5:00 p.m. (EST). E-mail address: docdelivery@haworthpress.com].

Available online at http://suba.haworthpress.com

doi:10.1300/J465v28n03_03

KEYWORDS. Alcohol, screening, substance abuse, brief intervention, SBIRT, drugs

INTRODUCTION

Screening, Brief Intervention, and Referral to Treatment (SBIRT) is a comprehensive, integrated, public health approach to the delivery of early intervention and treatment services for persons with substance use disorders, as well as those who are at risk of developing them. SBIRT is based on public health principles and procedures, and is designed to reduce the burden of injury, disease and disability associated with the misuse of psychoactive substances, particularly alcohol, illicit drugs, tobacco products, and prescription medications with high abuse potential. The aims of this review are to summarize the research base and state of knowledge on SBIRT. For the purposes of this review, the following are considered core components of SBIRT:

- *Screening:* SBIRT begins with the introduction of systematic screening into the normal routine at medical facilities and other community settings where persons with substance use disorders are likely to be found. Screening is by definition a preliminary procedure to evaluate the likelihood that an individual has a substance use disorder or is at risk of negative consequences from use of alcohol or other drugs. Whereas screening tests were initially developed to identify active cases of alcohol and drug dependence, in recent years the aim has been expanded to cover the full spectrum ranging from risky substance use to alcohol or drug dependence. Because the population of persons with risk factors is much larger than the population of dependence cases (1), SBIRT programs focusing on early intervention have generally adopted a broad definition of screening.
- *Brief intervention:* The term brief intervention refers to any time-limited effort (e.g., 1-2 conversations or meetings) to provide information or advice, increase motivation to avoid substance use, or to teach behavior change skills that will reduce substance use as well as the chances of negative consequences. Brief interventions are typically delivered to those individuals at low to moderate risk. Among the most cost-effective and time efficient interventions are brief motivational conversations between a health care professional and a substance user.
- *Brief treatment:* Brief treatment refers to the delivery of time-limited, structured (or specific) therapy for a substance use disorder by a trained clinician and is typically delivered to those at higher risk or in the early stages of dependence. It generally involves 2-6 sessions of cognitive-behavioral or motivational enhancement therapy with clients who are seeking help. Brief treatment may also include the ongoing management of substance use disorders in primary care settings, especially with the use of new pharmaceutical agents.
- *Referral to treatment:* Screening often identifies those who already have a substance-related health condition or a suspected substance use disorder that warrants a formal diagnosis and possible referral to treatment. The referral process facilitates access to care (including brief treatment) for those individuals who have more serious signs of substance dependence and require a level of care outside the scope of brief services.
- *Integration and coordination activities:* In many communities screening and brief intervention services are nonexistent, diagnostic and referral services are fragmented and inconsistent, and specialized treatment services operate independently of the larger health care system. A key aspect of SBIRT is the integration and coordination of these four components into a system of services linking the specialized treatment programs in a community with a network of early intervention and referral activities that are conducted in medical and social service settings.

As shown in Figure 1, SBIRT can be described as a set of inter-related services linked by decision rules that determine the appropriate course of action for a given patient. When risk is

FIGURE 1. SBIRT logic model

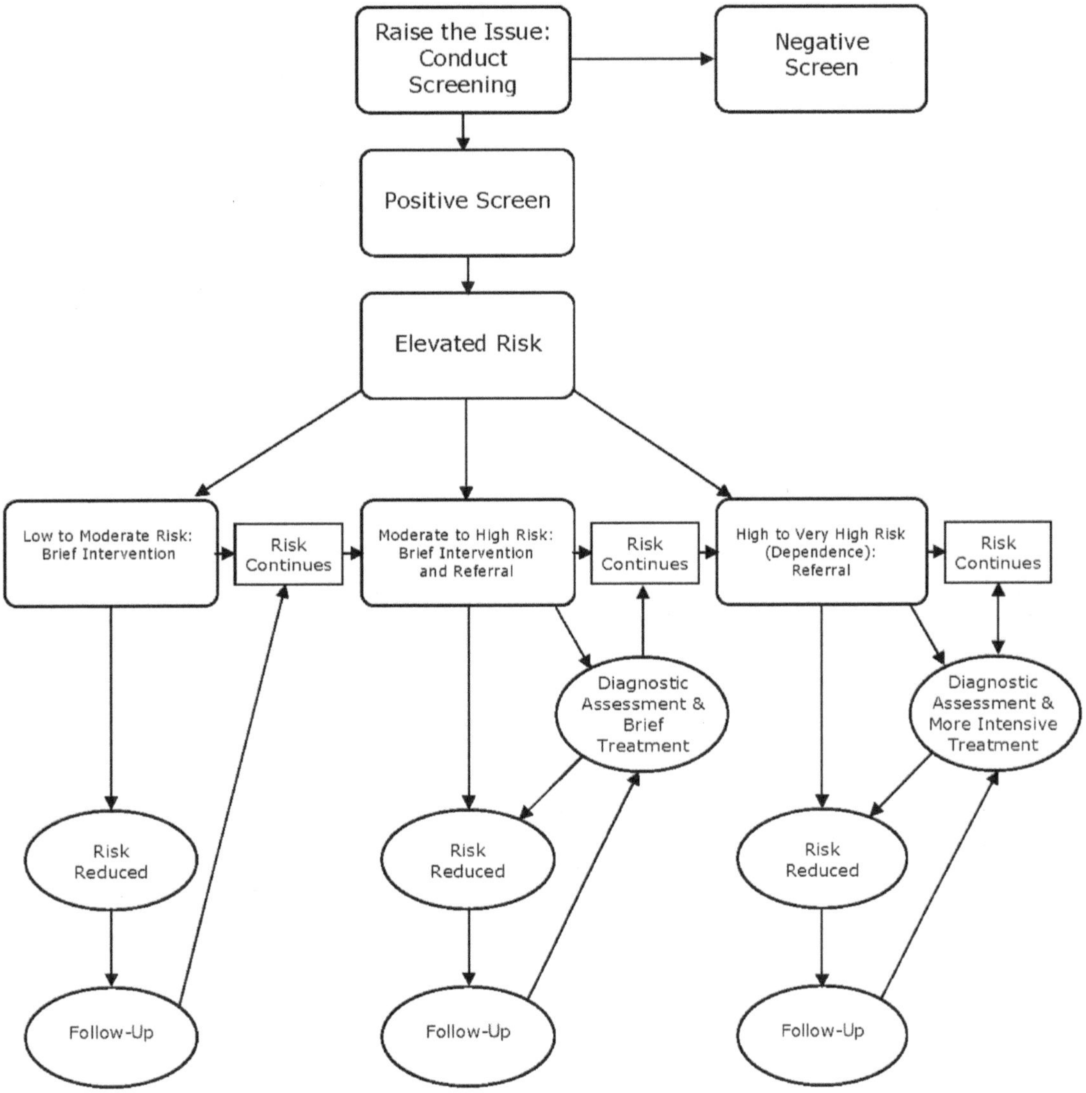

elevated but in the low range, brief intervention is the recommended course. Evidence is lacking regarding an exact cutoff for moderate risk, but several screening tests such as the AUDIT (2) have defined a mid-range of risk scores where further assessment, monitoring and brief treatment are warranted. Conceptually, anyone with elevated risk is eligible to begin with brief intervention even if the intent of the clinician is to deliver a referral to treatment or provide brief treatment. And in some cases, screening can lead directly to referral without feedback and advice. For those at low/moderate risk, the initial clinical procedure is brief intervention. For those at moderate or high risk, or with dependence, the goal would be a brief intervention that encourages entry into brief treatment or specialty treatment, respectively. Clearly many people at higher risk identified by screening will not receive specialty treatment. Follow-up ovals include arrows pointing back to the risk ovals in order to stress the need for continued monitoring and referral to further treatment if necessary.

The model for SBIRT is based in part on the Institute of Medicine (3) report that recommends the development of integrated service systems linking community-based screening and brief intervention with assessment and referral activities. One important function of SBIRT is to fill the gap between primary prevention efforts and more intensive treatment for persons with serious substance use disorders. From a public health perspective, the goal of SBIRT is to improve the health of a community by reducing the prevalence of adverse consequences of substance misuse, including but not limited to diagnosable abuse or dependence, through the coordination of early intervention and referral to specialized treatment. When all components are functioning effectively in health care and social service agencies throughout a community, SBIRT programs should be capable of reaching a significant proportion of the population using psychoactive substances.

A BRIEF HISTORY OF SBIRT

Although some SBIRT components date back as far as the early 18th century (4), it was not until the development of effective screening tests for alcohol and drug use in the 1980s that SBIRT emerged as a viable public health approach to addressing substance misuse. Screening instruments such as the MAST, the CAGE and the DAST were first developed to identify active cases of alcohol and drug dependence for referral to treatment (5). In the 1980s a seminal study by Russell et al. (6) showed how brief physician advice was capable of motivating small but significant numbers of patients to stop smoking. Subsequent research in Malmo, Sweden (7) indicated that systematic screening combined with brief interventions delivered in primary care settings were capable of reaching large numbers of at-risk drinkers, many of whom reduced their alcohol consumption in response to the program. The public health implications of the Malmo study for the prevention of alcohol problems led the World Health Organization (WHO) to initiate a program of clinical and applied research on the development of an international screening test and the evaluation of brief interventions for at-risk drinkers (8). That program, begun in 1981, led to the development of the Alcohol Use Disorders Identification Test (9) as well as the first cross-national clinical trial of the effectiveness of brief interventions in health care settings (10). The WHO program was expanded to include a consortium of researchers investigating ways to implement screening and brief intervention technologies in primary care settings, as well as the development of national plans to integrate SBIRT activities into the health care systems of both developed and developing countries (8). A related program was initiated in 1997 to develop a screening test and brief interventions for illicit drugs as well as alcohol and tobacco (11). These projects have been conducted during a 25-year period when there has been a dramatic increase in clinical and health services research on screening and brief intervention for alcohol and other substances. This research has been conducted primarily in the United States, Australia and European countries and has been accompanied by evaluations of training packages, implementation models, program costs and systems changes necessary to facilitate the adoption of SBIRT programs (2).

Perhaps the most significant development in this evidence-based movement to test and disseminate new screening and intervention technologies in the US is the Substance Abuse Mental Health Services Administration's SBIRT initiative, which consists of a variety of demonstration programs operating in 11 states. Other large scale programs have been implemented in Brazil, South Africa and the European Union. In the remainder of this review, we will critically evaluate the literature supporting the various components of SBIRT, summarizing this evidence in terms of its practical applications for program planners, administrators, and policymakers.

SCREENING

An important prerequisite for the SBIRT approach is the accurate identification of people at risk as well as active cases of substance abuse and dependence. Screening for alcohol, tobacco and other drugs has been gaining popularity in health care settings because of new technologies, expert committee recommendations and encouraging research findings about the effectiveness of early intervention (5,12,13). Table 1 provides a compendium of 25 self-report screening tests for alcohol and other substance use, abuse and dependence. The tests were identified in an extensive review of the literature published in peer reviewed journals covered in Index Medicus. For each screening test, the compendium lists the item content, target population, administration mode, number of items, scoring time, and the time frame of measurement. In this section, we update an evaluation of screening tests initially conducted by Babor and Kadden (5). Screening tests for alcohol and drugs are reviewed separately, and in both types of substances we further distinguish between self-report screening tests and biological tests that are conducted on samples of body fluids.

Alcohol screening tests: One of the first alcohol screening procedures, the Michigan Alcoholism Screening Test (MAST, 14), consists of 24 yes-no questions that list signs and symptoms of chronic alcoholism. The MAST has been criticized because of its length, its potential for falsification, and its focus on finding cases of alcohol dependence rather than early identification of risk factors. The shorter 12-item MAST (15) and the four-item CAGE screening test (16) increase the feasibility of screening but still maintain a focus on identifying active alcoholics. An added disadvantage of these screening tests is their use of questions measuring "lifetime" symptoms ("have you ever . . ."), which can produce false positives when the alcohol problems occurred in the past but have since remitted. A disguised screening test based on the patient's history of traumatic injury (17) was developed to deal with the falsification problem, but this was done at the expense of sensitivity and specificity.

A number of alcohol screening tests have been developed for special populations, including women (18,19) and the elderly (20). The World Health Organization developed the Alcohol Use Disorders Identification Test (AUDIT) (9,2) in order to maximize cultural and linguistic generalizability of screening results. The AUDIT focuses on both hazardous drinking as well as alcohol use disorders. The AUDIT has been well validated across different cultural groups in a variety of countries, and several shorter adaptations have been developed, including the AUDIT-PC, the AUDIT-FAST, and the AUDIT-C, all of which focus mainly on the quantity, frequency and pattern of drinking (21,22). Finally, several single item screening tests have been developed and validated. Williams and Vinson (23) found that a single question about the last episode of heavy drinking has good sensitivity and specificity in detecting hazardous drinking and alcohol use disorders. O'Brien et al. (24) found that by asking "How many days do you get drunk?" in a typical week, they could identify college students who are at higher risk of alcohol-related injury. To the extent that very short screening tests may motivate clinicians to screen more often, these tests may have value (see, for example, 25). Nevertheless, the value of longer tests is that the patient's responses to questions about drinking and alcohol problems can be the immediate point of departure for a brief intervention, which typically begin with a discussion of specific screening results.

Although not recommended for routine screening, several biological markers have been useful adjuncts to alcohol screening in emergency medicine and criminal justice settings, such as the breath alcohol concentration (BAC), gamma-glutamyltransferase (GGT, a liver enzyme), and carbohydrate-deficient transferrin (CDT). BAC has a short half-life and does not provide information about risk behavior other than to estimate the extent of recent drinking. GGT and CDT have not been found to be sensitive or specific enough to detect heavy episodic drinking (26).

Other psychoactive substances: Given the different needs and substance use patterns of adults and adolescents, self-report drug screening tests have generally been designed and validated for one or the other of these populations. Two types of self-report tests have been developed for adults. The first, exemplified by the Drug Abuse Screening Test (DAST; 27), consists of direct obvious or face valid questions about drug use and related problems that yields a quantitative score reflecting the severity of drug abuse. A later version of the DAST reduced the number of items from 28 to 10 without compromising reliability (28). In contrast to screening tests that ask directly about substance use, several tests have been developed to measure risk factors that are associated with actual or potential substance use disorders. However, tests of this type tend be quite long. For exam-

TABLE 1. Compendium of Alcohol and Drug Self-Report Screening Tests[a]

Name/Citation[b]	Content area[c]	Target Population[d]	Mode[e]	No. Items[f]	Admin. Time (minutes)	Scoring / interpret (minutes)	Time frame
AAIS Adolescent Alcohol Involvement Scale (135)	AP, AU, RF	adolescents	self	14	4	2 / minimal	Lifetime
ARPS Alcohol Related Problem Survey (136)	AP	elderly	self, interview	66	10	2 / also Computer	Past year
ASSIST Alcohol, Smoking, Substance Involvement Screening Test (11)	AP, AU, DP, DU	adults	interview	8	5	1/ minimal	Lifetime, past 90 days
AUDIT Alcohol Use Disorders Identification Test (2)	AP, AU	adults	self, interview	10	3/minimal	1/ minimal	Lifetime, past year
AUDIT – C	AP, AU	general	self, interview	3	1	1/minimal	Past year
AUDIT – FAST	AP, AU	general	self, interview	4	2	1/minimal	Past year
AUDIT – PC	AP, AU	general	self, interview	5	2	1/minimal	Past year
CAGE Cut Down, Annoyed, Guilty, Eye-Opener (16)	AP	general, elderly	self, interview	4	1.	1 /minimal	Lifetime
CAGE – AID (40)	AP, DP	general	self	4	1	1	Lifetime
CRAFFT Car, Relax, Alone, Friends, Forget, Trouble (39)	AP, AU, DP, DU	adolescents, young adults	self, interview	6	2/ minimal	1/minimal	Lifetime/Ever
CUGE Cut Down, Hurt Under Influence, Guilty, Eye-Opener (21)	AP, AU	college students	self	4	2	1/ minimal	Lifetime
DAST Drug Abuse Screening Test (28)	DP	general, Adolescents	self, Interview	28	5	1/ minimal	Lifetime
DUSI –R Drug Use Screening Inventory—revised (137)	AP, AU, DP, DU	adolescents, adults	self	159	20 – 40	15	Current, lifetime
FAST Fast Alcohol Screening Test (138)	AP, AU	general, emergency	interview	4	1	1	Past year
Five-Shot (139)	AP, AU	general, emergency	interview	5	5	5	Ever, current
MAST Michigan Alcoholism Screening Test (14)	AP	general	self, interview	25	5 /minimal	2 minimal	Lifetime

MSI-X Marijuana Screening Inventory (140)	DP.,DU	Adults	self, interview	31	5	1 minimal	Lifetime, past year, past month
POSIT Problem Oriented Screening Instrument for Teenagers (30)	AP,AU, DP, DU, RF	adolescents	self, interview, computer	139	20-30	2- 5	Lifetime, current
RAPS Rapid Alcohol Problems Screen (141)	AP	Emergency patients	self, interview	5	2 minimal	1 minimal	Past year
RUFT-Cut Riding, Unable to stop, Family & friends Trouble, Cut down (142)	AP, AU	adolescents, emergency	self, interview	5	1 minimal	1 minimal	Lifetime
SASSI Substance Abuse Subtle Screening Inventory (34)	AP, AU, DP, DU, RF	adults, adolescents	self, computer	93	15	5 also computer	Lifetime
SWAG Screening, Women, and Alcohol in Goteborg (143)	AP, AU	women	self	13	2 minimal	1 minimal	Ever
T-ACE Tolerance, Annoyed, Cut Down, Eye-Opener (144)	AP, AU	pregnant women	self, interview	4	2 minimal	1 minimal	Ever, current
Trauma Scale (27)	AP, RF	emergency	interview	4	1 minimal	1 minimal	Ever
TWEAK Tolerance, Worried, Eye-Opener, Amnesia, Cut down (19)	AU, AP	pregnant women	self, interview	5	2 minimal	1 minimal	Ever, current

[a] This table is an expanded and updated version of one previously published by Babor and Kadden (2005).

[b] Acronym or popular name is given first, followed by full name of test and primary source citation.

[c] The following content areas are coded where relevant: AU, alcohol use; DU, drug use; AP, alcohol problems; DP, drug problems; RF, risk factors.

[d] The primary target group for which the screening test was developed.

[e] Three modes of administration are coded: (1) self-report questionnaire (self); (2) interview; and (3) computer administration in the form of a self-report questionnaire.

[f] The number of items for three screening tests (DUSI, SASSI, POSIT) includes direct questions about substance abuse as well as scales measuring related risk factors.

ple, some of these tests are embedded in the Minnesota Multiphasic Personality Inventory, which contains over 500 items, and thus may not be appropriate to use in health care settings where there is limited time to administer and score the screening test (29).

Recognizing the need for a comprehensive screening and referral test for adolescents, the National Institute on Drug Abuse (NIDA) developed the Problem-Oriented Screening Instrument for Teenagers (POSIT) (30). The POSIT consists of 139 items that generate scores indicating problems in ten functional areas that are related directly or indirectly to substance use disorders: Substance Use/Abuse, Mental Health Status, Physical Health Status, Aggressive Behavior/Delinquency, Social Skills, Family Relations, Educational Status, Vocational Status, Peer Relations and Leisure and Recreation. The test has demonstrated good reliability and validity in adolescents referred to an assessment service for evaluation of substance use problems (31), but is too long to serve as a brief screening test. One option is to use only the Substance Use/Abuse part of the test, which would make it more efficient for screening in general health care settings.

In addition to the multidimensional screening approach used in the POSIT, several shorter instruments have been developed to screen specifically for substance use among adolescents. The Personal Experience Screening Questionnaire (PESQ) (32) focuses primarily on drug use and related problems, but also collects information on other areas of concern, such as psychopathology. Reliability and validity of this 38-item test have been demonstrated in the detection of individuals with different histories of substance use (33). Another adolescent screening test that has been used at adolescent treatment programs is the Substance Abuse Subtle Screening Inventory (SASSI, 34), a 78-item self-report instrument that classifies adolescents as chemically dependent. Although the SASSI was designed to prevent deliberate falsification by using indirect questions, it has not been found to be very accurate (35,36). Other screening tests have been designed for more specific populations, such as the 42-item Drug and Alcohol Problem (DAP) Quick Screen, which was developed for use by pediatricians (37). Validity data have been reported for the 30-item revision of this test (38). Finally, the CRAFFT (Car, Relax, Alone, Friends, Forget, Trouble) is brief (6 items) and has been validated with adolescents in primary care settings (39). Because of its brevity, it is more likely to be used than the longer instruments described above.

Combined screening tests: Despite advances in the development of self-report screening tests for specific types of psychoactive substances, there has been considerably less attention to instruments that screen for multiple substances. To address this deficiency, the Alcohol, Smoking and Substance Involvement Screening Test (ASSIST; 11) was developed to screen for at-risk use of psychoactive substances as well as related problems. The test uses a common format to screen for 11 psychoactive substances as well as injection drug use. The scoring procedure estimates the relative importance of these different risk behaviors for the purpose of prioritizing counseling interventions. Although the ASSIST is not able to identify people who exceed risky drinking limits based on quantities of alcohol consumed, these questions can easily be added to obtain country-specific alcohol risk levels.

A major challenge to combined screening for specific substances is provider burden, which refers to the skills and time demanded of the screening agent. A relatively simple procedure that addresses this problem is the CAGE test adapted to include drugs (CAGE-AID). The CAGE-AID was found to be more sensitive but less specific than the CAGE (40). This easy-to-use four-item test nevertheless requires further questioning if the patient scores positive. Thus, efficiency comes at the price of specificity, and screening questions using a lifetime (ever) approach can result in high numbers of false positives.

Biological Screening Methods for Drugs: A variety of biological procedures have been developed to detect recent drug use through urinalysis, hair testing, and saliva tests. These methods are not capable of detecting substance-related problems or even substance use beyond a narrow time window (41). Urine screening tends to be the preferred method because it is less invasive than blood testing and the drugs or their metabolites are present in relatively high concentrations in urine. A recent innovation that facilitates biological screening is the commercial availability of self-contained urine testing kits. These tests are easy to use and provide rapid access to test results, but they can only indicate drug use over the previous few days. Other problems include a risk of false positives by passive drug exposure or ingestion of foodstuffs, and false negatives due to the use of adulterants.

Summary: There are a number of important issues associated with screening instruments that should be taken into account in the design of an integrated SBIRT program intended to serve the needs of a defined population. First, the accuracy of most of the self-report tests has been evaluated under research conditions, which tend to maximize the likelihood of good performance. Although most screening tests have been found to be valid, performance is likely to diminish in routine clinical settings. A major concern is the extent to which the results of a self-report test can be deliberately faked or distorted in an attempt by the patient to preserve a respectable self-image in the health care or social service setting. Although self-report measures of substance use tend to be valid and reliable in the aggregate under most circumstances, accuracy in clinical settings depends on the degree of perceived threat in the data gathering situation, the cognitive processes (such as memory) that are required to produce answers to the questions, and the motivation and other personal characteristics of the respondent (42). A second consideration is cost and efficiency. Self-report tests are free or inexpensive, and they can be administered and scored quickly. Nevertheless, medical staff sometimes view even a small addition to their routine as an unnecessary burden. Although some screening tests are relatively brief (e.g., CAGE and AUDIT-C) and can be administered in one or two minutes, others require more time and administration skills. Biological tests can be costly to use on a routine basis and require even more time to administer and score. Nevertheless, they are often seen as being more consistent with routine medical practice, and this may affect their acceptability to both patients and staff. A third issue is cultural sensitivity. Although research has not been extensive, there is no evidence to suggest that the reliability or validity of self-report tests varies across different ethnic groups (9,11). A final issue is the target group of the screening program. Many of the adult screening tests described in Table 1 have been designed for finding active cases of alcohol or drug dependence, not to identify risk factors for drug or alcohol abuse. These tests (e.g., the DAST) typically avoid direct questions about use of specific drugs, focusing instead on the problems associated with any substance use in the past. Subtle or disguised screening tests (e.g., the SASSI) do not appear to be sufficiently sensitive or specific to identify active cases, but may be useful in screening for risk factors. Comprehensive screening tests like the POSIT and ASSIST are capable of identifying both "caseness" and risk factors, but they take more time to administer and score. Even single item or very brief screening tests like the AUDIT-C require further questioning once the patient screens positive, so screening tests with skip-out instructions like the AUDIT and ASSIST may save considerable time because most patients need not be screened further after negative responses to the first few questions.

BRIEF INTERVENTIONS

A key component of the SBIRT approach is the linking of screening results with appropriate early intervention services or referral to treatment. If intervention does not exist or is not feasible or effective, it is not useful to conduct screening. Among the least expensive interventions are brief motivational conversations between the substance user and a concerned physician, a nurse, a physician assistant or a social worker. In this section we review efficacy studies of brief interventions for excessive alcohol or drug use. Given the volume of research literature on this topic for alcohol, we will focus primarily on key studies and the results of meta-analyses of the cumulative literature. Brief interventions for drug use and abuse have been studied considerably less, so this literature is reviewed in terms of its preliminary findings and its deficiencies.

Brief interventions for alcohol abuse and at-risk drinking: In the first systematic review of research on this subject, Bien et al. (43) evaluated 32 controlled studies involving over 6000 patients studied prior to 1992. Brief interventions with problem drinkers were often found to be as effective as more extensive treatments. It was concluded that the course of harmful alcohol use can be effectively altered by relatively brief contacts in contexts such as primary health care settings and employee assistance programs. Kahan et al. (44) reviewed 11 trials of physician-based brief intervention in medical settings and concluded that brief alcohol interventions are effective, and their public health impact is potentially enormous. Twelve randomized controlled trials were reviewed by Wilk et al. (45), who concluded that brief intervention is a low-cost, effective preventive measure for heavy drinkers in outpatient settings. Additional support for these conclusions, based on new analyses of many of the same studies summarized in previous reviews, has been reported by Ballesteros et al. (46). Moyer et al. (47) reviewed studies comparing brief intervention both to untreated control groups and to more extended treatments. They found "further positive evidence" for the effectiveness of brief interventions, especially among patients with less severe problems. In an extensive review of the literature for the U.S. Preventive Services Task Force, Whitlock et al. (13) concluded that behavioral counseling interventions for alcohol misuse among nondependent primary care patients identified by screening are feasible and potentially effective components of an overall public health approach to reducing alcohol misuse.

Most of the studies cited in these reviews were conducted in primary care settings, where the prevalence of alcohol abuse and dependence tends to be lower than what is found in emergency and trauma centers. Emergency departments and trauma centers have been identified as high-yield settings for alcohol screening (12,48,49). A large randomized trial of brief interventions in a trauma center (50) found that a brief motivational intervention was associated with decreased alcohol consumption and a reduced risk of trauma recidivism.

In the course of investigating the efficacy of brief interventions with at-risk drinkers, research has also evaluated the extent to which behavior change is related to individual differences among drinkers, the professional training, ethnicity and gender of the intervention provider, and the nature of the intervention itself (13). In general, behavior change is not dependent on provider training or characteristics, but the dependence severity of the drinker does seem to be an important correlate of low response to brief intervention. Regarding the nature of the intervention, skills training, simple advice, and motivational approaches seem to be equally effective. In addition, the interventions seem to be equally effective with adolescents, adults, older adults, and pregnant women.

Despite the general preponderance of positive findings, some studies have shown no differences between intervention and control groups, and many studies report significant reductions in control group drinking that are comparable to those of the intervention group (51). One explanation for this phenomenon is that the screening procedure itself has a motivational effect, although one study found no evidence that assessment alone was responsible for changes in the control group (51). The other explanation is "regression to the mean," which describes a statistical tendency for extreme values such as heavy drinking to return to the group average over time.

Brief intervention for drug use and abuse: In contrast to the alcohol literature, there have been few studies of brief interventions for drug abuse. Bernstein et al. (52) found that brief intervention in a clinical setting can reduce cocaine and heroin use. Brief intervention appeared to facilitate abstinence at 6 months, even in the absence of meaningful contact with the treatment system. Baker et al. (53) found that both the provision of a self-help booklet and a single session of motivational interviewing were associated with reduced amphetamine consumption among regular users. Two studies (54,55) have found that general practitioners can reduce excessive benzodiazepine use in their patients using brief interventions such as letters or consultations. Despite these promising findings from controlled studies, and similar positive results from research described below under Brief Treatment, several investigators have reported negative findings from brief interventions with drug users. Marsden et al. (56) evaluated the effect of a stimulant-focused brief motivational interview (relative to the provision of health risk information about stimulants) among adolescent and young adult stimulant users. No significant differences between groups were found for ecstasy, powder cocaine, crack or alcohol. Other research (53) with psychiatric inpatients showed similar lack of effectiveness.

Summary: Research on brief interventions for alcohol and other substance users has accumulated rapidly during the past two decades. Not only are the procedures generally effective with a variety of population groups, they can be delivered with equal effect by a variety of health care providers. Less evidence is available regarding the brief interventions for drug users, but several studies show positive effects. An important question that requires further research is the extent to which brief interventions can be made more effective when combined with stepped care strategies that increase the intensity of the intervention for patients who do not respond initially. Among the options are brief treatment and referral to specialized programs serving persons with alcohol or drug dependence.

BRIEF TREATMENT

Brief treatment (BT) refers to the provision of as few as two sessions of therapy by a trained counselor, social worker, psychologist or psychiatrist. While brief interventions focus on motivating clients to change their substance use, brief treatment helps clients develop the skills and resources to change. BTs are often based on motivational approaches (e.g., Motivational Enhancement Therapy) or behavioral approaches (e.g., Cognitive-Behavioral Therapy) or a combination of the two. BT typically includes a standardized assessment procedure, goal-setting, and rapid implementation of change strategies. BT should be characterized as a self-contained modality, rather than fewer sessions of longer term or traditional therapy, or as more sessions of BI. The goals of BT differ from those of both longer term, traditional therapy and of BI. BT tends to focus on the present situation and emphasizes the use of effective therapeutic tools to make specific behavioral changes in a shorter period of time.

Studies have compared BT to more intensive, traditional treatment approaches and to BI approaches. Many have incorporated wait-listed control groups in the experimental design. Stephens, Roffman and Curtin (57) compared a brief, two-session individual treatment with 14 sessions of cognitive behavioral skills training. Both treatments produced substantial reductions in marijuana use relative to the delayed treatment control condition with treatment gains maintained at 16-month follow-up. The Marijuana Treatment Project (MTP) compared two treatment therapies with a delayed treatment control condition (58). One of the therapies consisted of nine individual counseling sessions delivered over a 12-week period. The other consisted of two motivational enhancement therapy sessions delivered over a one-month period. The nine-session intervention produced significantly greater reductions in marijuana use and associated consequences than the two-session intervention, and at each follow-up point over a 12-month period both treatments produced outcomes superior to the four-month delayed treatment control condition. The results indicate that even a brief two-session treatment is associated with substantial reductions in marijuana use and related problems in chronic marijuana users.

Several studies have demonstrated promising evidence that BT is often as effective as longer term, traditional therapies for substance use disorders (59-61). Moyer et al. (47) found positive evidence for the effectiveness of brief therapies, especially among patients with less severe problems. For clients with greater problem severity, Berglund et al. (62) noted that better results were observed with more treatment. Although studies show that patients who receive more outpatient mental health care tend to have better short-term substance use outcomes (63-65), there is growing evidence that duration and continuity of care is more important than the amount or intensity of care (66-69). The finding that duration of treatment (rather than amount of treatment) for alcohol and drug use disorders is more closely related to outcome suggests that more resources should be devoted to interventions such as brief treatments that are linked to other continuity of care options (70).

Summary: BT models are consistent with a public health approach in which large numbers of individuals at risk of developing serious alcohol or other drug problems may be identified through primary care screening or through court-mandated treatment (e.g., stemming from DUI arrests). The BT target population has traditionally been those individuals with less severe substance use disorders. However, there is a growing body of evidence to suggest that brief treatments are effective with a wide range of clients, including persons with mild to moderate alcohol dependence and regular marijuana users. BT may also be appropriate for some patients when previous attempts using traditional treatment approaches have failed, when there are insufficient resources (e.g., client time or insurance coverage) available for longer-term therapy, or when there are long waiting lists for specialized treatment. There is no question that BT is more effective than being on a waiting list and could benefit large numbers of clients who are seeking and waiting for longer term care (71).

MEDICATION-ASSISTED TREATMENT IN HEALTHCARE SETTINGS

Recent advances in pharmacological treatment for alcohol and opioid dependence provide significant opportunities to integrate the management of substance use disorders into primary health care. After screening and brief intervention, pharmacotherapy can be initiated in health care settings to assist patients undergoing BT or to facilitate the transition to traditional substance abuse treatment.

Medications for alcohol disorders: Four FDA-approved medications are available that physicians can prescribe to dampen craving, reduce heavy drinking, and/or promote abstinence. These are: naltrexone, a μ (mu)-opiate receptor antagonist; depot naltrexone, an extended-release form of naltrexone that is injected monthly; acamprosate calcium delayed-release tablets; and disulfiram (under supervised administration). These medications can be helpful to patients who are struggling to maintain sobriety and for preventing relapse after referral to treatment.

Of particular interest to SBIRT, one recent study looked at whether general internists and primary care physicians could treat alcohol-dependent patients as effectively as addiction specialists, using naltrexone (72). Results indicated that primary care counseling with naltrexone pharmacotherapy is a promising approach that can be effective in selected patients. In addition, the long acting, injectable form of naltrexone that is now available may enhance its use in primary care settings (73).

With the newer medications now available, there is increasing interest in whether alcohol-dependent individuals can be treated successfully with FDA-approved medications by their primary care physicians in routine medical practice. The comprehensive COMBINE clinical trial at 11 sites with nearly 1,400 patients explored a variety of treatment methods–alone and in combination–within the context of medical management (74). Alcohol consumption decreased by 80 percent over a 4-month treatment period, which suggests that medical management by primary physicians in routine practice can be of benefit in treating alcohol dependence (75). However, the medical management used in the COMBINE trial was relatively intensive (nine 20-minute sessions), so the minimal level of contact with primary care physicians necessary to manage alcohol-dependent patients has not yet been determined.

The COMBINE Study also found that naltrexone in combination with a brief behavioral therapy delivered by licensed health care professionals is more effective than more intensive behavioral therapy delivered by licensed behavioral health specialists (74).

Medications for drug dependence: The Drug Addiction Treatment Act of 2000 established a new paradigm for the medication-assisted treatment of opioid dependence. Qualifying physicians in a medical office or other appropriate settings may now apply to the Substance Abuse and Mental Health Services Administration (SAMHSA) to prescribe and/or dispense opioid medications for treating opioid addiction. Two sublingual formulations of buprenorphine, a long-acting partial agonist of mu-opioid receptors, have been approved by the FDA for this purpose.

The decision to allow office based treatment of buprenorphine was based on a large body of clinical experience from other countries and the United States (76-78). A Cochrane Review meta-analysis of 13 randomized clinical trials concluded that buprenorphine is an effective intervention for use in the maintenance treatment of heroin dependence (79).

REFERRAL TO ASSESSMENT AND SPECIALIZED SUBSTANCE ABUSE TREATMENT

Research suggests that brief intervention alone may not be sufficient therapy for severely dependent drinkers (80). Because many brief intervention trials specifically exclude people dependent on alcohol or drugs, it is not known whether this population may be helped by brief interventions alone. Thus, for patients with severe conditions, SBIRT programs need to make referrals to more intensive treatment and to mutual support groups such as Alcoholics Anonymous (AA), Narcotics Anonymous (NA), and Cocaine Anonymous (CA).

Research demonstrates that hospital patients identified as substance dependent during medical screening (most of whom are not seeking treatment) can be effectively referred and engaged in specialized treatment at rates much greater than controls (81-85). In these individual program studies, brief interventions have increased the percent of patients who show up for their first clinic appointment from 5 percent among controls to from 50 to 65 percent, with as many as 50 percent of patients reporting that they continue to be involved in some kind of substance abuse treatment or 12-step meetings on follow-up (81-83).

Information is limited about the prognosis for alcohol- and drug-dependent patients seen and referred in other medical settings, where patients are highly heterogeneous in terms of type, stage, and severity of substance problems, with many of these patients not motivated to start treatment (86). Prognosis appears to be strongly related to the patient's motivation to enter treatment, as well as to change drinking or drug-using behavior (85).

The literature provides little information about the specific referral processes used by various SBIRT programs. However, existing evidence suggests that brief motivational interventions have positive benefit on patients' participation in substance abuse treatment and retention in treatment. For example, when one hospital replaced staff referrals with motivational interview techniques done by alcohol specialists, the percent of referred patients who completed treatment increased from 40 to 88 percent (85). In another study, 65 percent of patients who received a brief motivational intervention kept their initial interview at an alcohol clinic, compared to 5.4 percent of the control group (83).

These findings indicate that SBIRT referral methods need to address the patient's motivation to be treated, with the added intention of reducing the risk of drop-out and assisting the patient's adherence to treatment. Based on the available literature, it is not possible to say which brief intervention approaches, in which settings, and with which patients will be most effective for promoting entry and engagement into specialized alcohol or drug treatment. The research shows that the earlier substance-dependent patients engage in treatment or mutual-help groups, the better the outcomes (87,88).

IMPLEMENTATION, INTEGRATION AND COORDINATION ACTIVITIES

A major challenge to the public health impact of SBIRT is the difficulties involved in integrating its components into relevant parts of the health care system.

Screening: As noted above, progress has been made in the development of a variety of effective screening procedures. Nevertheless, a number of practical and logistical issues need to be resolved before a screening program can be implemented. These issues relate not only to who does the screening, but when, where, how often and who pays for it. Given the simplicity of most self-report screening tests, they are capable of being administered in variety of different settings and modalities, such as interview, questionnaire, and computer. Dyches et al. (89) describe an interactive telephone technology for screening with primary care patients. Both patients and practitioners had rated the procedure positively. Under some circumstances, impersonal procedures, such as paper and pencil questionnaires and computer-assisted telephone interviews, may be more effective than face-to-face interviews with physicians. Saitz et al. (90) report 50,000 visits a year for screening at an internet web site where positive cases received advice and information, suggesting that an accessible web site can attract high risk drinkers for screening and brief intervention.

In the absence of routine screening with standardized instruments, physicians do not systematically apply NIAAA guidelines regarding hazardous drinking levels (91) and may be selective in whom they screen. One study (92) found that physicians were least likely to initiate discussions about drinking with patients who are white, female and widows. A Danish study of screening by general practitioners (93) reported that physicians did not think all patients should be screened. The major barriers were lack of time and financial incentives, and skepticism that patients wanted to be screened.

Some investigators (94) have argued that primary health care is not an effective or efficient place to conduct alcohol screening. Others have suggested alternative sites for screening and professionals who can conduct it. Anderson et al. (95) identified the clergy as potential providers of screening and brief intervention. Hungerford et al. (96) report that screening in an emergency department can produce high rates of acceptance of counseling about alcohol use. In a rural university emergency department (12), only 3% of the patients screened or counseled were uncooperative; 70% thought the emergency department was a good place to help patients with alcohol problems. Another potential setting for screening programs is trauma centers. Schermer et al. (97) found that 70% of trauma patients were successfully screened, with less than 1% refusing. Nevertheless, a survey (98) of 50 insurance commissioners indicated 38 states where there are concerns about the possibility that screening will affect insurance payments, which can be denied in many states if the patient has been drinking.

Brief intervention: According to Roche and Freeman (99), physician-based secondary prevention efforts based on brief interventions for hazardous drinking have failed at the implementation stage. Barriers to implementation include lack of time, poor diagnostic skills, negative attitudes, and perceptions of role incompatibility (100). In a survey of 711 trauma surgeons (97), 83% agreed that the trauma center was an appropriate setting but only 25% used formal screening questionnaires and less than one half of problem patients are addressed in their hospital stay. Barriers included cost, time, confidentiality and threats to insurance coverage.

To overcome some of these barriers, other delivery agents (e.g., nurses) have been considered. D'Onofrio and Degutis (101) describe the use of non-physician health promotion advocates (HPAs) to do SBI and referrals in the emergency department.

Another way to expand the use of brief interventions is through internet applications. A review of the small number of web-based interventions (102) found that a demand does seem to exist for this kind of service and the potential impact could be considerable. As noted above, Saitz et al. (90) recorded 50,000 screening visits a year at an internet web site. Positive cases received advice and information, suggesting that an accessible web site can attract high-risk drinkers for brief interventions.

Another barrier to brief intervention is competition for the provider's time once a patient screens positive. Saitz et al. (103) showed that the very act of screening can prompt physicians to increase discussions and provide advice. Brady et al. (104) found that prompting of providers using other means doubled the rate of brief intervention. In a study by Kaner et al. (105), patient and practitioner characteristics predicted who got a brief intervention after screening: males, the unemployed, and technically trained workers were more likely to receive an intervention than females and employed persons. In addition, practitioners with more training and longer practice experience were more likely to deliver interventions. Babor et al. (106,107) compared two different implementation strategies for Cutting Back, a primary care alcohol screening and brief intervention program for hazardous and harmful drinkers. In one model, medical providers were responsible for delivering interventions. In another model mid-level professionals (usually nurses) acted as the clinic specialists to provide that service. In a sample of 10 health clinics, the mid-level professionals screened a higher percentage of patients than did the medical providers during the best month of program operation (50% vs. 44%) and over all months of operation (24% vs. 19%). Of those patients who screened positive, more patients screened by the mid-level professionals received an intervention than in the provider model (73.1% vs. 57.1%).

The ability of clinics to conduct SBI was significantly correlated with both staffing characteristics and organizational factors (e.g., prior experience, organizational stability, number of clinicians trained and the quality of the coordinator's work). Lack of time, staff turnover and competing priorities correlated negatively with SBIRT implementation.

In summary, the primary obstacles to the use of SBIRT in applied settings are: (1) lack of time for overburdened health care workers; (2) training and motivation of professionals to administer screening and intervention to at-risk drinkers; and (3) organizational factors including administrative support and competing priorities. Successful implementation of the technology tends to occur at those sites where clinicians are reimbursed for their services and are well trained for the task. In addition, the extent to which a given delivery model is likely to work best within a managed care organization depends on complex provider and organizational characteristics.

Brief treatment: Although there are insufficient data to determine which populations might benefit most from Brief Treatment, a growing literature suggests that BT is effective with a wide range of substance abusing clients. Further, the majority of clients receiving substance abuse treatment stay in therapy for relatively short periods of time (between 6 and 20 one-hour sessions). Although this statistic argues for a greater use of structured BT approaches in current clinical practice, DHHS (71) found that many therapists trained in traditional approaches were resistant to using structured BT models. A related problem is that brief treatment is typically developed, evaluated and delivered in an individual therapy format, whereas traditional treatment tends to be offered in group format because of cost considerations.

The demonstration of several efficacious brief treatment interventions, especially for marijuana dependence, raises questions about how best to engage chronic marijuana users in treatment and how best to maintain improvements following treatment. Unfortunately, very little research has been conducted in these areas. A pilot study was conducted to evaluate a program designed to offer a guided self-assessment (but not treatment) to persons interested in changing their marijuana use. It successfully used a variety of recruitment strategies to attract participants, including posters, radio and newspaper ads, and outreach at various community events (108). The check-up program offered a useful method for reaching non-treatment-seeking heavy marijuana users, and at follow-up program participants reported a significant reduction in the frequency of marijuana use when compared to those who just got information. These results suggest that standalone programs that provide discrete treatment to regular marijuana users may be feasible and can reach large numbers of clients if they are properly designed and advertised.

Training and technology transfer: Training in how to conduct screening and brief interventions is clearly a vital component in assuring effective implementation of SBIRT components. Introducing new screening and prevention activities into primary care practices and other settings presents significant challenges to professional training and continuing education. Medical schools and residency programs devote limited faculty resources and curriculum time to substance abuse (109-111) and many professionals feel inadequately trained when faced with patients who have substance-related problems (112,113). Barriers to adequate coverage of alcohol and drug-related problems in both medical schools and continuing professional education include traditional attitudes about the moral culpability of chronic alcoholics, confusion as to whether problem drinking is a medical or psychiatric concern, lack of faculty role models, lack of training materials, and role ambiguity regarding who is responsible for screening and intervention (114,115). Research on medical education has shown that training can be effective in improving students' and physicians' knowledge and skills in addressing alcohol issues (106, 116-118), but changes in knowledge may be easier to produce than changes in attitudes and behavior (119). A review of the components and outcomes of medical education in substance-related disorders concluded that the selection of a combined didactic and interactive educational strategy may be the most cost-effective learning strategy, but there is little empirical evidence to support this approach (119).

Although some progress has been made in the development of SBIRT for medical practitioners, medical students, and health care organizations (1,120,121), a necessary step toward dissemination is the development of successful training packages that include program implementation procedures. Babor et al. (106) found that following a relatively short (3-hour) workshop and subsequent supervision, physicians experienced an increased sense of confidence in performing screening procedures. In addition, non-physician clinicians perceived fewer obstacles to screening patients after receiving the training. When delivered in the context of a comprehensive SBIRT implementation program, training was effective in changing providers' knowledge, attitudes, self-efficacy and practice of screening and brief interventions for at-risk drinking. The results are consistent with other studies of provider behavior (116,122, 123) which show that health care providers trained to deliver a brief alcohol intervention will counsel their at-risk patients when cued to do so and when supported by a primary care office system. Adams et al. (123) found that a 2.5-hour training doubled the rate of alcohol interventions in high-risk primary care patients. Wilk and Jensen (124) used standardized patients (i.e., actors who play the role of symptomatic patients) to train residents to use SBI. After training more residents conducted screening and brief interventions. Gomel et al. (125) compared three strategies to market and train primary care physicians. Tele-marketing was more cost-effective than academic detailing and direct mail in promoting uptake of an SBI package. Roche et al. (117) compared two educational programs to train medical students; interactive training was no more effective than traditional didactic lectures in developing knowledge and skills. These studies suggest that SBIRT training can be effective in providing skills, increasing self-efficacy, and changing provider behavior.

In summary, training programs have been developed and adapted to specialty settings (e.g., physicians in primary care clinics). Educational materials for use with problem drinkers have also been developed. Manuals, pamphlets, and books have been written to help train professionals in the process of SBI. Research on all of these training packages suggests that they increase knowledge about drug misuse, but they vary in their ability to change provider behavior. More research is needed on how increased knowledge translates into behavior changes and what factors help to sustain those behavior changes.

ECONOMIC CONSIDERATIONS

There are several important economic issues to consider in relation to implementing SBIRT. Providers, financial managers, and decision makers need accurate information about the costs of screening and brief interventions and estimates of the revenue potential. Decision makers also need to know the cost-effectiveness of various SBIRT models in order to choose between lower cost/less effective models and higher cost/more effective models. Cost benefit estimates are needed to assess the net costs to health plans or to society of diverting resources to SBIRT activities. In this section we summarize research on each of these issues.

Cost: SBIRT costs will vary, depending on the perspective from which costs are calculated, e.g., the provider's, the payer's, the patient's, or society's perspective. For financial management purposes, the total costs of SBIRT services can be broken down into their components, e.g., screenings, information packets, counseling sessions, and case management. From the *provider's perspective* the cost of brief interventions depends primarily on the nature and severity of the client's alcohol or drug problems, the number of sessions that comprise the interventions, the personnel delivering brief interventions, the resources to produce and deliver interventions (and treatments) and the settings in which brief interventions are provided. Providers must also consider the one-time costs of developing and starting the service plus any on-going continuing costs such as continuing education of staff. From the *client's perspective,* the cost of SBIRT includes the amount the client pays for the intervention beyond the premiums for health insurance, as well as time and transportation costs to the site where interventions are furnished. From *a payer's perspective,* the cost of brief interventions might be defined as the amount paid for the service minus any financial benefit that may accrue from the reduction of future costs resulting from the service. From *society's perspective,* the cost of brief interventions is expressed in terms of the market value of the best alternative use to which labor, capital, and other resources may be put (i.e., economic or opportunity costs).

Given the various perspectives that could be used, it is not surprising that published estimates of the costs of SBIRT vary considerably. For example, Zarkin et al. (126) estimated screening costs at $0.42 per patient for a 2-minute screen versus $16 per patient by Gentilello et al. (127) and $497 per patient by Kunz et al. (128). Given the fact that fewer than 30 percent of patients screened are referred for brief interventions, efforts to reduce the initial screening costs can significantly reduce the overall cost of providing alcohol SBI. There is also broad variability in the costing methodology used in the literature. For example, brief intervention costs have been reported at $2.59 per patient (126), $135 per brief intervention session (128), and $0.59 median per member per month (insurance premium cost) (129). Obviously, the underlying variability of the SBI programs is a primary cause for the variation in cost estimates, but the lack of a consistent costing methodology contributes to the variability and limits the usefulness of cross-program comparisons.

Furthermore, current SBI cost-effectiveness and cost-benefit research often presents cost results without a detailed description of the costing methods used. Many of these studies do not adequately address how and what was actually costed (e.g., 130). Authors often take national wage averages and estimate the amount of time for services (e.g., 127). The most thorough cost estimate comes from the Cutting Back study (126), which used activity-based costing to separate start-up costs from ongoing implementation costs, a distinction overlooked by previous studies. Cutting Back is the only study to compare costs across providers and is also the first to cost different models of implementation. However, the SBI models studied by Zarkin et al. (126) were implemented exclusively for the Cutting Back research project, and therefore the authors were forced to make judgments as to which costs would likely be retained in a non-research setting.

Cost effectiveness analysis: Cost effectiveness analysis (CEA) enables decision makers to compare the economic merits of alternative types of service, such as brief interventions and standard care, which represents the care that clients would ordinarily receive. Kunz et al. (128) found cost-effectiveness ratios for brief interventions administered in a hospital emergency department of $258 for a one unit reduction in the follow-up AUDIT score, $219 for a decrease of one drink per week, and $61 for a one percentage point decline in the follow-up probability of heavy drinking. In a study that applied estimates from published studies to Australia, Wutzke et al. (130) found that brief physician advice to at-risk drinkers resulted in additional years of life from fewer accidents. Dividing the cost of the intervention by the number of life-years saved yielded a cost of approximately Aus $1,873 per life-year saved. CEA does not, however, provide definitive recommendations on which program should be adopted. Rather, it provides decision makers with evidence on the relative benefits and costs of one program compared to another. For this reason, CEA alone is often not enough to justify adoption of a new program.

Cost benefit analysis: Unlike CEA, CBA places a dollar value on all outcomes and directly compares to the dollar value of a program's outcomes to the dollar value of its costs. As a result, CBA often provides definitive answers on which programs should be adopted. The program with the largest dollar benefit after accounting for costs should unambiguously be adopted. There are various methods with which to compare the benefits of a program to its costs, including: net benefit measures in which costs are subtracted from benefits; return on investment in which the benefits are expressed as a percentage return to the investment represented by the program costs; and the benefit cost ratio in which benefits are expressed as a ratio of the costs. The choice of CBA measure is largely determined by the audience, with return on investment often appealing more to business or corporate audiences and net benefit or benefit-cost ratios appealing more to academic audiences.

The CBA evidence on SBIRT is generally very favorable. In a randomized trial of brief interventions administered in physician offices, Fleming and colleagues (131) found that a group receiving a brief intervention not only had significant reductions in alcohol use, they also had fewer hospital days and fewer emergency department visits. The intervention cost $205 per person ($166 from the clinic perspective and $39 from the client's perspective) and saved $712 in health care costs. The benefit cost ratio of 4.3 suggests a $43,000 savings in future health care costs for every $10,000 spent for early intervention. The benefit cost ratio increased to 39:1 after factoring fewer motor vehicle and legal events into the analysis.

In a CBA using published sources, Gentilello et al. (127) estimated that the screening and brief alcohol interventions provided to injured patients treated in an emergency department or admitted to a hospital together cost $54 per patient, or $16 plus $38, respectively. The net cost savings from the screening and intervention was estimated at $89 per patient, or $330 for each patient receiving an intervention (27 percent had a positive screen). The benefit, in the form of reduced direct health costs, resulted in a savings of $3.81 for every $1.00 spent on screening and intervention, for a benefit cost ratio of 3.8:1. If interventions were routinely offered to injured adult patients nationwide, it was estimated that the potential net savings might approach $1.82 billion annually.

In a retrospective study of admissions to the Naval Medical Center in Portsmouth, Virginia, Storer (132) estimated that intervention patients had significantly lower hospital readmission rates than other patients. The lower readmission rate for intervention patients alone generated an estimated savings of $606,400, for a total cost of $31,500 (benefit cost ratio of 19:1), for an average cost of $154 for 205 brief interventions.

Summary: Although the findings support the use of certain SBIRT components on economic grounds, the studies should be used cautiously. The cost effectiveness of SBIRT may vary considerably, depending on how the technology is applied. If a program is aimed at a selected, high-risk portion of the population (e.g., emergency room patients with injury or trauma), a higher rate of risky drinkers will be identified than in a "population approach" (e.g., all members of an HMO), where a cross-section of the entire population is screened (133). This issue will affect the rate at which people receive an SBIRT service and the economic efficiency of any such operation. Similarly, the potential for cost savings is much greater among a higher risk portion of the population. The labor cost of personnel designated to screen and conduct brief intervention, and whether SBIRT is their sole function or is incorporated into other functions will affect cost effective calculations. Additionally, the extent of the intervention–whether one five-minute session at the time of the screening, or multiple sessions of longer duration on different days–will significantly affect both treatment costs and costs incurred by patients.

CONCLUSION: TRANSLATING RESEARCH INTO PRACTICE

In the parlance of contemporary medical science, "translation" has three inter-related meanings: (1) applying what we have learned from research to practical settings; (2) making scientific knowledge accessible and relevant to practitioners; and (3) improving the health of the population by broad dissemination of effective medical and health promotion technologies. Translation from research to practice can be considered at two levels: (1) from the laboratory "bench" to the patient's "bedside"; and (2) from bedside to the entire community. In the former (called T1 translation), basic science research leads to new clinical investigation and interventions. Examples of T1 bench to bedside applications from the 25 years of SBIRT research considered in this review include the discovery of biomarkers for alcohol and drug screening, the use of psychometric theory to develop new self-report screening tests, and the development of new medications to dampen alcohol craving, reduce heavy drinking, and/or promote abstinence. Examples of the second form of translation, where clinical investigation leads to improved medical practice and enhanced population health (called T2 translation), are studies of SBIRT training, program implementation and cost effectiveness. Although much work needs to be done at both T1 and T2 levels, the findings of this review indicate that significant progress has been made in translating research into practice. For example, since 1980:

- Several hundred empirical studies on screening, brief intervention, referral and integration of SBIRT into health care settings have been conducted.
- Over 25 screening tests have been developed and validated.
- Scores of randomized controlled trials of brief intervention have been conducted in a wide range of countries.
- 15 or more integrative reviews of the SBIRT literature have been published.
- A growing literature on provider training, SBIRT implementation, and new applications is now available.

Based on the results of this review, the following conclusions seem warranted about the various components of SBIRT:

- Self-report screening tests are reliable and valid under most clinical conditions, but the use of screening tests depends on provider and patient characteristics.
- Self-report response bias can be predicted, detected and minimized.
- Brief Interventions (BI) can reduce alcohol use for at least 12 months in non-dependent heavy drinkers.
- The approach is acceptable to both genders and to adolescents and adults.
- Cost-effectiveness has been demonstrated in several countries.
- Brief interventions are effective with smokers and risky drinkers, and there is some evidence that they work well with marijuana users.
- Brief treatments are effective with persons who are dependent on alcohol, marijuana or other drugs.
- SBIRT risk reduction materials exist in diverse formats.

After two decades of clinical research, program development and evaluation studies, SBIRT is poised for the next step in dissemination. There is general agreement on the need to "broaden the base" of treatment by expanding SBIRT services to less severe cases and populations at risk. In order for this to happen, the traditional, acute care model of curative medicine will have to be expanded to include a new population-based healthcare management perspective in which persons experiencing or at risk of substance use disorders are provided with a range of preventive, curative, and rehabilitative services. These services should be designed to fit the needs of defined populations, with providers organized into networks that attempt to shift utilization to lower cost settings or most appropriate level of care. Implementation models are currently inadequate to achieve sufficient population reach unless routine screening, which is the linchpin of SBIRT, is organized throughout the health care and social service systems. Contractual models for screening, brief intervention, and referral may work better in settings where there are limited resources or staff resistance. In all cases, it is important to fit the SBIRT program to the population, rather than requiring that patients suit the needs of the providers. It is clear from the findings of this review as well as other research (134) that population-wide measures to implement the various SBIRT components could have a significant effect on reducing the burden of illness associated with substance use disorders.

Nevertheless, there are still gaps in the literature, which suggest the need for further research. Little research has been devoted to the potential role that SBIRT could play to increase access to treatment for people with alcohol and drug dependence. Additional research is needed to evaluate screening and brief intervention methods for illicit drug users in general medical settings. To the extent that SBIRT programs are part of a broader network of specialized and general health care services, research is need to determine how best to implement SBIRT programs, how to evaluate their impact on indicators of population health (such as alcohol-related morbidity and drunk driving rates), and what are the costs and benefits to society.

REFERENCES

1. Babor TF, Higgins-Biddle JC. Alcohol screening and brief intervention: Dissemination strategies for medical practice and public health. *Addiction*. 2000;95: 677-86.

2. Babor TF, Higgins-Biddle JC, Saunders JB, Monteiro MG. *AUDIT The Alcohol Use Disorders Identification Test: Guideline for Use in Primary Care*. 2nd ed. Geneva: World Health Organization; 2001.

3. Institute of Medicine. *Broadening the Base of Treatment for Alcohol Problems*. Washington DC: National Academies Press; 1990.

4. Babor TF. Avoiding the "horrid and beastley sin of drunkenness:" Does dissuasion make a difference? *J Consult Clin Psychol*. 1994;62:1127-1140.

5. Babor TF, Kadden RK. Screening and interventions for alcohol and drug problems in medical settings: What works? *J Trauma*. 2005;59(3 Suppl):S80-S87.

6. Russell MA, Stapleton JA, Hajek P. District programme to reduce smoking: Can sustained intervention by general practitioners affect prevalence? *J Epidemiol Community Health*. 1988;42:111-115.

7. Kristenson H, Ohlin H, Hulten-Nosslin B, Trell E, Hood B. Identification and intervention of heavy drinking in middle aged men: Results and follow-up of 24-60 months of long-term study with randomized controls. *Alcohol Clin Exp Res*. 1983;7:203-209.

8. Babor TF, de la Fuente JR, Saunders J, Grant M. *AUDIT The Alcohol Use Disorders Identification Test: Guidelines for Use in Primary Health Care*. WHO/MNH/DAT 89.4. Geneva: World Health Organization; 1989.

9. Saunders JB, Aasland OG, Babor TF, de la Fuente JR, Grant M. Development of the Alcohol Use Disorders Identification Test (AUDIT): WHO collaborative project on early detection of persons with harmful alcohol consumption-II. *Addiction*. 1993;88:791-804.

10. WHO Brief Intervention Study Group. A cross national trial of brief intervention with heavy drinkers. *Am J Public Health*. 1996;86:948-955.

11. WHO ASSIST Working Group. The Alcohol, Smoking and Substance Involvement Screening Test (ASSIST): Development, reliability and feasibility. *Addiction*. 2002;97:1183-1194.

12. Hungerford DW, Pollock DA. Emergency department services for patients with alcohol problems: Research directions. *Acad Emerg Med*. 2003;10:79-84.

13. Whitlock EP, Polen MR, Green CA, Orlean T, Klein J. Behavioral counseling interventions in primary care to reduce risky/harmful alcohol use by adults: A summary of the evidence for the US Preventive Services Task Force. *Ann Intern Med*. 2004;140:557-568.

14. Selzer ML. The Michigan Alcoholism Screening Test: The quest for a new diagnostic instrument. *Am J Psychiat*. 1971;127:1653-1656.

15. Selzer ML, Vinokur A, Van Rooijen L. A self-administered Short Michigan Alcoholism Screening Test (SMAST). *J Stud Alcohol*. 1975;36:117-126.

16. Ewing JA. Detecting alcoholism: The CAGE questionnaire. *JAMA*. 1984;252:1905-1907.

17. Skinner HA, Holt S. Identification of alcohol abuse using laboratory tests and a history of trauma. *Ann Intern Med*. 1984;101:847-851.

18. Russell M. New assessment tools for risk drinking during pregnancy: T-ACE, TWEAK, and others. *Alcohol Health Res World*. 1994;18:55-61.

19. Chan AW, Pristach EA, Welte JW, Russell M. Use of the TWEAK test in screening for alcoholism/heavy drinking in three populations. *Alcohol Clin Exp Res*. 1993;17:1188-1192.

20. Moore AA, Beck JC, Babor TF, Hays RD, Reuben DB. Beyond alcoholism: Identifying older, at-risk drinkers in primary care. *J Stud Alcohol*. 2002; 63: 316-324.

21. Aertgeerts B, Buntinx F, Bande-Knops J, Vandermeulen C, Roelants M, Ansoms S, Fevery J. The value of CAGE, CUGE, and AUDIT in screening for alcohol abuse and dependence among college freshmen. *Alcohol Clin Exp Res*. 2000;24:53-57.

22. Canagasaby A, Vinson D. Screening for hazardous or harmful drinking using one or two quantity-frequency questions. *Alcohol Alcohol*. 2005;40:208-213.

23. Williams R, Vinson DC. Validation of a single screening question for problem drinking. *J Fam Pract*. 2001;50:307-312.

24. O'Brien MC, McCoy TP, Champion H, et al. Single question about drunkenness to detect college students at risk for injury. *Acad Emerg Med*. 2006;13: 629-636.

25. Vinson DC, Galliher JM, Reidinger C, Kappus JA. Comfortably engaging: which approach to alcohol screening should we use? *Ann Fam Med*. 2004;2: 398-404.

26. Peterson K. Biomarkers for alcohol use and abuse–A summary. *Alcohol Res Health*. 2004;28(1): 30-37.

27. Skinner HA. The Drug Abuse Screening Test. *Addict Behav*. 1982;7:363-371.

28. Gavin DR, Ross HE, Skinner HA. Diagnostic validity of the drug abuse screening test in the assessment of DSM-III drug disorders. *Br J Addict*. 1989;84: 301-307.

29. Greene RL, Weed NC, Butcher JN, Arredondo R, Davis HG. A cross-validation of MMPI-2 substance abuse scales. *J Pers Assess*. 1992;58:405-410.

30. Rahdert E. *The Adolescent Assessment and Referral Manual*. DHHS Publication No. ADM-91-1735. Rockville, MD: National Institute on Drug Abuse; 1991.

31. McLaney MA, Del Boca FK, Babor TF. A validation study of the problem-oriented screening instrument for teenagers. *J Mental Health*. 1994;3:363-376.

32. Winters K. *Manual for the Personal Experience Screening Questionnaire (PESQ)*. Los Angeles: Western Psychological Services; 1990.

33. Winters KC. Development of an adolescent alcohol and other drug abuse screening scale: Personal experience screening questionnaire. *Addict Behav*. 1992;17: 479-490.

34. Miller FG. SASSI: Application and assessment for substance-related problems. *Subst Use Misuse*. 1997;2:163-166.

35. Feldstein SW, Miller WR. Does subtle screening work? A review of the SASSI. *Addiction*. 2007;102: 41-50.

36. Svanum S, McGrew J. Prospective screening of substance dependence: The advantages of directness. *Addict Behav*. 1995;20:205-213.

37. Klitzner M, Schwartz RH, Gruenewald P, Blasinsky M. Screening for risk factors for adolescent alcohol and drug use. *Am J Dis Child.* 1987;141:45-49.

38. Schwartz RH, Wirtz PW. Potential substance abuse: Detection among adolescent patients: Using the drug and alcohol problem (DAP) quick screen, a 30-item questionnaire. *Clin Pediatr.* 1990;29:38-43.

39. Knight JR, Shrier LA, Bravender TD, Farrell M, Vander Bilt J, Shaffer HJ. A new brief screen for adolescent substance abuse. *Arch Pediatr Adolesc Med.* 1999;153:591-596.

40. Brown RL, Rounds LA. Conjoint screening questionnaires for alcohol and other drug abuse: Criterion validity in a primary care practice. *Wis Med J.* 1995;94:135-140.

41. Wolff K, Farrell M, Marsden J, Monteiro MG, Ali R, Welch S, Strang J. A review of biological indicators of illicit drug use, practical considerations and clinical usefulness. *Addiction.* 1999;94:1279-1298.

42. Babor TF, Brown J, Del Boca F. Validity of self-reports in applied research on addictive behaviors: Fact or fiction. *Behav Assess.* 1990;12:5-31.

43. Bien T, Miller WR, Tonigan JS. Brief interventions for alcohol problems: A review. *Addiction.* 1993;88:315-336.

44. Kahan M, Wilson L, Becker L. Effectiveness of physician-based interventions with problem drinkers: A review. *Can Med Assoc J.* 1995;152:851-859.

45. Wilk AI, Jensen NM, Havighurst TC. Meta-analysis of randomized control trials addressing brief interventions in heavy alcohol drinkers. *J Gen Intern Med.* 1997; 12(5):274-283.

46. Ballesteros J, Duffy JC, Querejeta I, Arino J, Gonzalez-Pinto A. Efficacy of brief interventions for hazardous drinkers in primary care: Systematic review and meta-analyses. *Alcohol Clin Exp Res.* 2004;28: 608-618.

47. Moyer A, Finney J, Swearingen C, Vergun P. Brief interventions for alcohol problems: A meta-analytic review of controlled investigations in treatment-seeking and non-treatment seeking populations. *Addiction.* 2002;97:279-292.

48. Gentilello, LM, Rivara FP, Donovan DM, Dunn CW, Rivera FP. Alcohol interventions in trauma centers. *JAMA.* 1995;274:1043-1048.

49. Charalambous MP. Alcohol and the accident and emergency department: A current review. *Alcohol Alcohol.* 2002;37:307-312.

50. Gentilello LM, Donovan DM, Dunn CW, Rivara FP. Alcohol interventions in a trauma center as a means of reducing the risk of injury recurrence. *Ann Surg.* 1999;230:1-18.

51. Daeppen JB, Gaume J, Bady P, et al. Brief alcohol intervention and alcohol assessment do not influence alcohol use in injured patients treated in the emergency department: A randomized controlled clinical trial. *Addiction.* 2007;120(8):1024-1033.

52. Bernstein E, Bernstein J, Tassiopoulos K, Heeren T, Levenson S, Hingson R. Brief intervention at a clinic visit reduced cocaine and heroin use. *Drug Alcohol Depend.* 2005;77:49-59.

53. Baker A, Lee NK, Claire M, Lewin TJ, Grant T, Pohlman S. Brief cognitive behavioural interventions for regular amphetamine users: A step in the right direction. *Addiction.* 2005;100:367-378.

54. Cormack MA, Sweeney KG, Hughes-Jones H, Foot GA. Evaluation of an easy, cost-effective strategy for cutting benzodiazepine use in general practice. *Br J Gen Pract.* 1994;44:5-8.

55. Bashir K, King M, Ashworth M. Controlled evaluation of brief intervention by general practitioners to reduce chronic use of benzodiazepines. *Br J Gen Pract.* 1994;44:408-412.

56. Marsden J, Stillwell G, Barlow H, Boys A, Taylor C, Hunt N, Farrell M. An evaluation of a brief motivational intervention among young ecstasy and cocaine users: no effect on substance and alcohol use outcomes. *Addiction.* 2006;101(7):1014-1026.

57. Stephens RS, Roffman RA, Curtin L. Comparison of extended versus brief treatments for marijuana use. *J Consult Clin Psychol.* 2000;68:898-908.

58. Marijuana Treatment Project Research Group. Brief treatments of cannabis dependence: Findings from a randomized multi-site trial. *J Consult Clin Psychol.* 2004;72:455-466.

59. McLellan AT, Arndt ID, Metzger DS, Woody GE, O'Brien CP. The effects of psychosocial services in substance abuse treatment. *JAMA.* 1993;269(15): 1953-1959.

60. Gottheil E, Weinstein SP, Sterling RC, Lundy A, Serota RD. A randomized controlled study of the effectiveness of intensive outpatient treatment for cocaine dependence. *Psychiatr Serv.* 1998;49:782-787.

61. Miller WR, Hester RK. Treating alcohol problems: Toward an informed eclecticism. In: Hester RK, Miller WR, eds. *Handbook of Alcoholism Treatment Approaches: Effective Alternatives,* 3rd ed. Boston: Allyn & Bacon; 2003.

62. Berglund M, Thelander S, Salaspuro M, Franck J, Andreasson S, Ojehagen A. Treatment of alcohol abuse: An evidence-based review. *Alcohol Clin Exp Res.* 2003;27:1645-1656.

63. Fiorentine R, Anglin D. More is better: Counseling participation and the effectiveness of outpatient drug treatment. *J Subst Abuse Treat.*1996;13:341-348.

64. Brochu S, Slandry M, Bergeron J, Chiocchio F. The impact of a treatment process for substance users as a function of their degree of exposure to treatment. *Subst Use Misuse.* 1997;32:1993-2011.

65. Jerrell JM, Ridgely MS. The relative impact of treatment program "robustness" and "dosage" on client outcomes. *Eval Program Plann.* 1999;22:323-330.

66. Ouimette PC, Moos RH, Finney JW. Influence of outpatient treatment and 12-step involvement on one-year substance abuse treatment outcomes. *J Stud Alcohol.* 1998;59(5):513-522.

67. Moos RH, Finney JW, Federman EB, Suchinsky R. Specialty mental health care improves patients' out-

comes: Findings from a nationwide program to monitor the quality of care for patients with substance use disorders. *J Stud Alcohol.* 2000;61(5):704-713.

68. Ritsher J, Finney J, Moos R. The influence of treatment orientation and continuing care on substance abuse patients' two-year remission. *Psychiatr Serv.* 2002;53:595-601.

69. Moos RH. Addictive disorders in context: Principles and puzzles of effective treatment and recovery. *Psychol Addict Behav.* 2003;17(1):3-12.

70. Humphreys K, Tucker J. Toward more responsive and effective systems for alcohol-related problems. *Addiction.* 2002;97:126-132.

71. Department of Health and Human Services, Substance Abuse and Mental Health Services Administration. *Brief Interventions and Brief Therapies for Substance Abuse, Treatment Improvement Protocol* (TIP) No 34. Rockville, MD: Center for Substance Abuse Treatment; 1999.

72. O'Malley SS, Rounsaville BJ, Farren C, Namkoong K, Wu R, Robinson J, O'Connor PG. Initial and maintenance naltrexone treatment for alcohol dependence using primary care vs specialty care: A nested sequence of 3 randomized trials. *Arch Intern Med.* 2003;163:1695-1704.

73. Johnson BA, Ait-Daoud N, Aubin HJ, Van Den Brink W, Guzzetta R, Loewy J, Silverman B, Ehrich E. A pilot evaluation of the safety and tolerability of repeat dose administration of long-acting injectable naltrexone (Vivitrex) in patients with alcohol dependence. *Alcohol Clin Exp Res.* 2004;28:1356-1361.

74. Anton RF, O'Malley SS, Ciraulo DA, Cisler RA, Couper D, Donovan DM, Gastfriend DR, Hosking JD, Johnson BA, LoCastro JS, Longabaugh R, Mason BJ, Mattson ME, Miller WR, Pettinati HM, Randall CL, Swift R, Weiss RD, Williams LD, Zweben A, for The COMBINE Study Research Group. Effect of combined pharmacotherapies and behavioral interventions (The COMBINE Study) for alcohol dependence. *JAMA.* 2006;295:2003-2017.

75. Kranzler HR. Evidence-based treatments for alcohol dependence: New results and new questions. *JAMA.* 2006;295:2075-2076.

76. Ling W, Wesson DR. Clinical efficacy of buprenorphine: Comparisons to methadone and placebo. *Drug Alcohol Depend.* 2003;70(2Suppl):S49-S57.

77. Bridge TP, Fudala PJ, Herbert S, Liederman DB. Safety and health policy considerations related to the use of buprenorphine/naloxone as an office-based treatment for opiate dependence. *Drug Alcohol Depend.* 2003;70(2Suppl):S79-S85.

78. Amass L, Ling W, Freese TE, Reiber C, Annon JJ, Cohen AJ, McCarty D, Reid MS, Brown LS, Clark C, Ziedonis DM, Krejci J, Stine S, Winhusen T, Brigham G, Babcock D, Muir JA, Buchan BJ, Horton T. Bringing buprenorphine-naloxone detoxification to community treatment providers: The NIDA Clinical Trials Network Field Experience. *Am J Addict.* 2004;13:S42-S66.

79. Mattick RP, Kimber J, Breen C, Davoli M. *Buprenorphine maintenance versus placebo or methadone maintenance for opioid dependence.* The Cochrane Database of Systematic Reviews 2003; Issue 2, pub2: CD002207.

80. Fleming MF, Graham AW. Screening and brief interventions for alcohol use disorders in managed care settings. *Recent Dev Alcohol.* 2001;15:393-416.

81. Bernstein E, Bernstein J, Levenson S. Project ASSERT: An ED-based intervention to increase access to primary care, preventive services, and the substance abuse treatment system. *Ann Emerg Med.* 1997;30: 181-189.

82. D'Onofrio G, Bernstein E, Bernstein J, Woolard RH, Brewer PA, Craig SA, Zink BJ. Patients with alcohol problems in the emergency department, part 2: Intervention and referral. SAEM Substance Abuse Task Force. Society for Academic Emergency Medicine. *Acad Emerg Med.* 1998;5:1210-1217.

83. Dunn CW, Ries R. Linking substance abuse services with general medical care: Integrated, brief interventions with hospitalized patients. *Am J Drug Alcohol Abuse.* 1997;23:1-13.

84. Elvy GA, Wells, JE, Baird KA. Attempted referral as intervention for problem drinking in the general hospital. *Br J Addict.* 1988;83:83-89.

85. Hillman A, McCann B, Walker NP. Specialist alcohol liaison services in general hospitals improve engagement in alcohol rehabilitation and treatment outcome. *Health Bulletin.* 2001;59:420-423.

86. Rochat S, Wietlisbach V, Burnand B, Landry U, Yersin B. Success of referral for alcohol dependent patients from a general hospital: Predictive value of patient and process characteristics. *Subst Abus.* 2004;25(1): 9-15.

87. Timko C, Moos RH, Finney JW, Moos BS, Kaplowitz MS. Long-term treatment careers and outcomes of previously untreated alcoholics. *J Stud Alcohol.* 1999;60:437-447.

88. Moos RH, Moos BS. Long-term influence of duration and intensity of treatment on previously untreated individuals with alcohol use disorders. *Addiction.* 2003;98(3):325-337.

89. Dyches H, Alemagno S, Llorens SA, Butts JM. Automated telephone-administered substance abuse screening for adults in primary care. *Health Care Manag Sci.* 1999;2:199-204.

90. Saitz R, Larson MJ, Horton NJ, Winter M, Samet JH. Linkage with primary medical care in a prospective cohort of adults with addictions in inpatient detoxification: Room for improvement. *Health Serv Res.* 2004;39(3):587-606.

91. Spandorfer JM, Israel Y, Turner BJ Primary care physicians' views on screening and management of alcohol abuse: Inconsistencies with national guidelines. *J Fam Pract.* 1999;48(11):899-902.

92. Arndt S, Schultz SK, Turvey C, Petersen A. Screening for alcoholism in the primary care setting:

Are we talking to the right people? *J Fam Pract.* 2002;51:41-46.

93. Hansen LJ, de Fine ON, Beich A, Barfod S. Screening for alcohol overconsumption in general practice. Experiences of general practitioners with a patient questionnaire. *Ugeskr Laeger.* 2001;163:2358-2361.

94. Beich A, Thorsen T, Rollnick S. Screening in brief intervention trials targeting excessive drinkers in general practice: Systematic review and meta-analysis. *BMJ.* 2003;327:536-542.

95. Anderson PA, Grey SF, Nichols C, Parran TV Jr, Graham AV. Is screening and brief advice for problem drinkers by clergy feasible? A survey of clergy. *J Drug Educ.* 2004;34:33-40.

96. Hungerford DW, Pollock DA, Todd KH. Acceptability of Emergency Department-based screening and brief intervention for alcohol problems. *Acad Emerg Med.* 2000;7:1383-1392.

97. Schermer CR, Bloomfield LA, Lu SW, Demarest GB. Trauma patient willingness to participate in alcohol screening and intervention. *J Trauma.* 2003;54(4): 701-706.

98. Rivara FP, Tollefson S, Tesh E, Gentilello LM. Screening trauma patients for alcohol problems: Are insurance companies barriers? *J Trauma.* 2000;48(1): 115-118.

99. Roche AM, Freeman T. Brief interventions: Good in theory but weak in practice. *Drug Alcohol Rev.* 2004;23(1):11-18.

100. Modesto-Lowe V, Boornazian A. Screening and brief intervention in the management of early problem drinkers: Integration into healthcare settings. *Disease Management & Health Outcomes.* 2000;8(3):129-137.

101. D'Onofrio G, Degutis LC. Preventive care in the Emergency Department: Screening and brief intervention for alcohol problems in the Emergency Department: A Systematic Review. *Acad Emerg Med.* 2002; 9:627-638.

102. Copeland J, Martin G. Web-based interventions for substance use disorders: A qualitative review. *J Subst Abuse Treat.* 2004;26:109-116.

103. Saitz R, Horton N J, Sullivan LM, Moskowitz MA, Samet JH. Addressing alcohol problems in primary care: a cluster randomized, controlled trial of a systems intervention. The Screening and Intervention in Primary Care (SIP) study. *Ann Intern Med.* 2003;138(5):372-382.

104. Brady M, Sibthorpe B, Bailie R, Ball S, Sumnerdodd P. The feasibility and acceptability of introducing brief intervention for alcohol misuse in an urban aboriginal medical service. *Drug Alcohol Rev.* 2002;21:375-380.

105. Kaner EFS, Healther N, Brodie J, Lock CA, McAvoy BR. Patient and practitioner characteristics predict brief alcohol intervention in primary care. *Br J Gen Pract.* 2001;51:822-827.

106. Babor TF, Higgins-Biddle JC, Higgins P, Gassman R, Gould B. Training medical providers to conduct alcohol screening and brief intervention. *Subst Abus.* 2004;25(1):17-26.

107. Babor TF, Higgins-Biddle J, Dauser, Higgins P, Burleson J. Alcohol screening and brief intervention in primary care settings: Implementation models and predictors. *J Stud Alcohol.* 2005;66:361-369.

108. Stephens RS, Roffman RA, Burke R, Williams C, Balmer A, Picciano J, Adams S. *"The Marijuana Check-Up."* Paper presented at the annual conference of the Association of Behavior Therapy, Washington, DC; November 1998.

109. Fleming MF, Barry KL, Davis A, Kahn R, Rivo M. Faculty development in addiction medicine: Project SAEFP, a one-year followup study. *Fam Med.* 1994; 26:221-225.

110. Brewster J, Single E, Ashley M, Chow YC, Skinner H, Rankin M. Preventing alcohol problems: Survey of Canadian medical schools. *Can Med Assoc J.* 1990; 143:1076-1082.

111. Fleming MF, Manwell LB, Barry KL, Adams W, Stauffacher EA. Brief physician advice for alcohol problems in older adults: A randomized community-based trial. *J Fam Pract.* 1999;48(5):378-384.

112. Wallace P, Haines A. The use of a questionnaire in general practice to increase the recognition of patients with excessive alcohol consumption. *BMJ.* 1985; 90(6486):1949-1953.

113. Church OM, Babor TF. Barriers and breakthroughs: Substance abuse curricula in nursing education. *J Nurs Educ.* 1995;34:278-281.

114. Negrete JC. The role of medical schools in the prevention of alcohol-related problems. *Can Med Assoc J.* 1990;143(10):1048-1053.

115. Bendtsen P, Akerlind I. Changes in attitudes and practices in primary health care with regard to early intervention for problem drinkers. *Alcohol Alcohol.* 1999;34:795-800.

116. Ockene JK, Adams A, Hurley TG, Wheeler EV, Hebert JR. Brief physician- and nurse practitioner-delivered counseling for high-risk drinkers: Does it work? *Arch Intern Med.* 1999;159(18):2198-2205.

117. Roche AM, Stubbs JM, Sanson-Fisher RW, Saunders JB. A controlled trial of educational strategies to teach medical students brief intervention skills for alcohol problems. *Prev Med.* 1997;26(1):78-85.

118. Walsh RA, Sanson-Fisher RW, Low A, Roche AM. Teaching medical students alcohol intervention skills: Results of a controlled trial. *Med Educ.* 1999; 33(8):559-565.

119. El-Geubaly N, Toews J, Lockyer J, Armstrong S, Hodgins D. Medical education in substance-related disorders: Components and disorders. *Addiction.* 2000;95: 949-957.

120. McRee B. Curriculum for Implementing Screening and Brief Intervention Services for Smokers and At-risk Drinkers in Primary Care Settings. Robert Wood Johnson's Prescription for Health Toolkit 2004. Available at: http://www.prescriptionforhealth.org/toolkit/index.html.

121. Richmond R, Heather N, Wodak A, Kehoe L, Webster I. Controlled evaluation of a general prac-

tice-based brief intervention for excessive drinking. *Addiction.* 2000;95(6):949-957.

122. McRee B, Granger J, Babor TF, Feder I, Folino M, Horn A, Steinberg J, vom Eigen K Reducing tobacco use and risky drinking in underserved populations: The need for better implementation models. *Ann Fam Med.* 2005;3(2):558-560.

123. Adams A, Ockene JK, Wheller EV, Hurley TG. Alcohol counseling: Physicians will do it. *J Gen Intern Med.* 1998;13:692-698.

124. Wilk AI, Jensen NM. Investigation of a brief teaching encounter using standardized patients: Teaching residents alcohol screening and intervention. *J Gen Intern Med.* 2002;17(5):356-360.

125. Gomel MK, Wutzke SE, Hardcastle DM, Lapsley H, Reznick RB. Cost-effectiveness of strategies to market and train primary health care physicians in brief intervention techniques for hazardous alcohol use. *Soc Sci Med.* 1998;47:203-211.

126. Zarkin GA, Bray JW, Davis KL, Babor TF, Higgins-Biddle JC. Costs of screening and brief intervention for risky alcohol use. *J Stud Alcohol.* 2003;64: 849-857.

127. Gentilello LM, Ebel BE, Wickizer TM, Salkever DS, Rivara FP. Alcohol interventions for trauma patients treated in emergency departments and hospitals: A cost benefit analysis. *Ann Surg.* 2005;241:541-550.

128. Kunz FM, French MT, Bazargan-Hejazi S. Cost-effectiveness analysis of a brief intervention delivered to problem drinkers presenting at an inner-city hospital emergency department. *J Stud Alcohol.* 2004;65: 363-370.

129. Broskowski A, Smith S. *Estimating the Cost of Preventive Services in Mental Health and Substance Abuse Under Managed Care.* DHHS Pub. No. SMA-02-3617. Rockville, MD: SAMHSA; 2001.

130. Wutzke SE, Shiell A, Gomel MK, Conigrave KM. Cost effectiveness of brief interventions for reducing alcohol consumption. *Soc Sci Med.* 2001;52:863-870.

131. Fleming MF, Mundt MP, French MT, Manwell LB, Staauffacher EA, Barry KL. Brief physician advice for problem drinkers: Long-term efficacy and cost-benefit analysis. *Alcohol Clin Exp Res.* 2002;26:36-43.

132. Storer RM. A simple cost-benefit analysis of brief interventions on substance abuse at Naval Medical Center Portsmouth. *Mil Med* .2003;168(9):765-768.

133. NIAAA. *Eighth Special Report to the U.S. Congress on Alcohol and Health by NIAAA.* September 1993. Table 5, P.14.

134. Chisholm D, Rehm J, Van Ommeren M, Monteiro M. Reducing the global burden of hazardous alcohol use: A comparative cost-effectiveness analysis. *J Stud Alcohol.* 2004;65:782-793.

135. Mayer J, Filstead WJ. The Adolescent Alcohol Involvement Scale: An instrument for measuring adolescents' use and misuse of alcohol. *J Stud Alcohol.* 1979;40:291-300.

136. Fink A, Morton SC, Beck JC, Hays R, Spritzer K, Tsai M, Moore AA. Comparing the alcohol-related problems survey (ARPS) to traditional alcohol screening measures in elderly outpatients. *Arch Gerontol Geriatr.* 2002;34:55-78.

137. Tarter RE. Evaluation and treatment of adolescent substance abuse: A decision tree method. *Am J Drug Alcohol Abuse.* 1990;16:1-46.

138. Hodgson R, Alwyn T, John B, Thom B, Smith A. The FAST Alcohol Screening Test. *Alcohol Alcohol.* 2002;37:61-66.

139. Seppa K, Lepisto J, Sillanaukee P. Five-shot questionnaire on heavy drinking. *Alcohol Clin Exp Res.* 1998;22(8):1788-1791.

140. Alexander DA. Marijuana Screening Inventory (Experimental Version): Description and preliminary psychometric properties. *Am J Drug Alcohol Abuse.* 2003;29(3):619-645.

141. Cherpitel CJ. Screening for alcohol problems in the emergency room: A rapid alcohol problems screen. *Drug Alcohol Depend.* 1995;40:133-137.

142. Kelly TM, Donovan JE, Chung T, Cook RL, Delbridge TR. Alcohol use disorders among emergency department-treated older adolescents: A new brief screen (RUFT-Cut) using the AUDIT, CAGE, CRAFFT, and RAPS-QF. *Alcohol Clin Exp Res.* 2004;28:746-753.

143. Spak F, Hallstrom T. Screening for alcohol dependence and abuse in women: Description, validation, and psychometric properties of a new screening instrument, SWAG, in a population study. *Alcohol Clin Exp Res.* 1996;20(4):723-731.

144. Sokol RJ, Martier SS, Ager JW. The T-ACE questions: Practical prenatal detection of risk-drinking. *Am J Obstet Gynecol.* 1989;160(4):863-870.

doi:10.1300/J465v28n03_03

ASSESSMENT: HOW IT WORKS

Methodological Issues in Alcohol Screening and Brief Intervention Research

Kypros Kypri, PhD

SUMMARY. The research literature on screening and brief intervention (SBI) for unhealthy alcohol use is large and diverse. More than 50 clinical trials and 9 systematic reviews have been published on SBI in a range of healthcare settings, and via a variety of delivery approaches, in general practice, hospital wards, emergency departments, addiction treatment centres, and more recently, via computers and the Internet. The aim of this paper was to discuss methodological issues which arise in the design, analysis, interpretation, and reporting of SBI trials. Principal among these are the challenge of detecting small effects, standards of analysis, reporting, and interpretation, the risks of bias arising from self-report of outcomes, and the need to ensure that results have the potential to be applied in practice to reduce the burden of disease and injury attributable to unhealthy alcohol use. doi:10.1300/J465v28n03_04 *[Article copies available for a fee from The Haworth Document Delivery Service: 1-800-HAWORTH. E-mail address: <docdelivery@haworthpress.com> Website: <http://www.HaworthPress.com> © 2007 by The Haworth Press, Inc. All rights reserved.]*

KEYWORDS. Methodology, trial, screening, brief intervention, alcohol, drinking

INTRODUCTION

A significant advance in the treatment of unhealthy alcohol use has been the development of screening and brief intervention (SBI). SBI typically involves opportunistic administration by a physician or nurse of a brief screening questionnaire such as the AUDIT (1) and, for

Kypros Kypri is affiliated with the School of Medicine and Public Health, University of Newcastle, Australia, Injury Prevention Research Unit, University of Otago, New Zealand.

Address correspondence to: Kypros Kypri, School of Medicine and Public Health, University of Newcastle, Australia, David Maddison Building, cnr King & Watt Streets, Newcastle NSW 2300 Australia (E-mail: kypros.kypri@newcastle.edu.au).

The author gratefully acknowledges the Stichting Volksbond Rotterdam and the Addiction Research Institute Rotterdam for the IVO award, which facilitated his writing of this paper, and insightful comments on a draft manuscript from Professor Richard Saitz.

[Haworth co-indexing entry note]: "Methodological Issues in Alcohol Screening and Brief Intervention Research." Kypri, Kypros. Co-published simultaneously in *Substance Abuse* (The Haworth Medical Press, an imprint of The Haworth Press, Inc.) Vol. 28, No. 3, 2007, pp. 31-42; and: *Alcohol/Drug Screening and Brief Intervention: Advances in Evidence-Based Practice* (ed: Richard Saitz, and Marc Galanter) The Haworth Medical Press, an imprint of The Haworth Press, Inc., 2007, pp. 31-42. Single or multiple copies of this article are available for a fee from The Haworth Document Delivery Service [1-800-HAWORTH, 9:00 a.m. - 5:00 p.m. (EST). E-mail address: docdelivery@haworthpress.com].

Available online at http://suba.haworthpress.com

doi:10.1300/J465v28n03_04

those who screen positive, provision of 5-10 minutes brief advice or a brief session (usually < 30 minutes) of motivational therapy (2). Where there are severe problems or alcohol dependence is suspected, a referral may be made for further assessment and specialist treatment (3). More than 50 clinical trials have been published on SBI, many of which have been conducted in primary healthcare settings (4). The results of seven systematic reviews show that 15 minutes of SBI produces modest but clinically meaningful reductions in alcohol consumption and related problems of 6-12 months among persons not actively seeking treatment for a drinking problem (4,5). Their use in primary healthcare is now recommended by health authorities in several countries, including the USA (6).

Although the evidence for its efficacy is strong, SBI is still not routinely offered in primary healthcare in any country. This is not because of a lack of staff knowledge or skill, but rather, practitioners' concerns about damaging rapport with patients, and their notions of role legitimacy. For example, Beich and colleagues (7) report that many GPs are reluctant to initiate discussion about alcohol with patients through fear of damaging rapport, and Lock et al. (8) found that many medical practice staff do not see screening as a legitimate part of their role.

Even if all primary care practitioners did routinely implement SBI, some patients have little or no contact with primary care settings, or are reluctant to acknowledge problems in a face-to-face interaction. There is a need for alternative methods to complement traditional face-to-face intervention, e.g., via the use of computers, and therefore a need for further clinical trials to determine the efficacy of such approaches. As the effort to provide an evidence base for practice increases, it is important that it benefits from the experience of more than 20 years of research on more traditional methods of SBI. This paper canvasses some methodological issues which researchers may wish to consider in the design, analysis and reporting of studies concerning SBI.

DESIGN ISSUES

Sample size. Relative to clinical trials of other interventions used in primary healthcare, e.g., pharmacotherapy for hypertension [e.g., (9)], which typically involve many thousands of patients, the brief intervention literature is comprised of mainly small studies, usually including only a few hundred participants, with some trials including fewer than 30 persons per arm.

The expected effect sizes of brief intervention are modest, its virtue lying in the aggregation of effects across a large portion of the population, afforded by low implementation cost per unit of intervention. The propensity to conduct small studies creates a high risk of Type II error, i.e., the failure to detect treatment effects due to insufficient statistical power. Conversely, the review process may be subject to the risk of *publication bias* (10), i.e., the tendency for under-powered clinical trials with statistically significant findings, some of which reflect Type I error, to be more often reported in the scientific literature than studies with non-significant results (11). Large meta-analytic reviews like that conducted by Moyer et al. can identify publication bias by pooling the results with and without the smaller trials (5). Notably, in the recent systematic review of brief intervention trials by Bertholet et al., studies judged to be of lower overall quality, appeared to bias results toward the null, rather than away from it, i.e., better studies were more likely to find that brief intervention produced positive effects (4).

Assessment effects. Assessment is a foundation of all clinical practice for the purpose of diagnosis, treatment planning, and monitoring outcomes. The methodological implications of a patient's drinking improving without subsequent intervention has stimulated much speculation and some research (12,13). The methodological challenges relate primarily to the blurring of experimental contrast when assessment has a therapeutic benefit, which is particularly important for an intervention whose therapeutic benefits are modest at the individual level. Assessment effects can be considered a source of contamination, and present a significant challenge for the field, described thus by Clifford and Maisto (14), in their review of assessment effects research:

> The disentangling of research and treatment effects is critical if research is to im-

> prove decisions made about alcohol treatment. The separation of subject reactivity and treatment effects is essential, to the degree that it is present in the typical randomized controlled trial (RCT), because most people presenting for alcohol treatment are never exposed to the research component. (p. 787).

A recent RCT of web-based SBI (15) explored the concept that assessment of patients' drinking risk status without subsequent intervention might have beneficial effects. In a university student health service, 975 patients (17-29 years) completed a web-based AUDIT questionnaire. Of 599 who scored ≥ 8 (mean 15.0, SD 5.2), 576 consented to follow-up and were included in a four-arm trial, of whom 293 (153 women) were assigned to either a group which received an information leaflet at baseline, or a group which received the information leaflet and 10 min of web-based assessment 4 weeks later. A year after baseline, relative to the leaflet only group, those who received web-based assessment reported significantly lower overall consumption (−18%), fewer heavy drinking episodes (−34%), fewer problems (−19%), and lower AUDIT scores (−1.6 points). These results suggest that in many SBI trials, results may be biased toward the null because of assessment effects.

Measuring outcome. It is common for hazardous drinkers to intersperse periods lasting days and weeks, in which they consume little or no alcohol, with bouts of very heavy consumption. Other unhealthy use may be characterised by sustained heavy consumption. Intervention may, if effective, produce yet more variability in these distributions of alcohol consumption. Capturing and analysing this variability is a significant challenge in clinical trials. Some studies assess an entire 12 months' alcohol consumption, relying on patient accounts of typical drinking frequency and quantity, an approach which often fails to take account of occasional very heavy episodes. Less commonly, data are collected regularly (e.g., monthly), creating a large response burden and accentuating the problems of missing data and attrition. Many studies focus on a single point in time, e.g., one month drinking reported at a 12 month follow-up time point, which has the advantage of not placing excessive demands on recall, but the disadvantage of missing earlier effects or variations in the 11 months of data not counted. There are no fix all solutions to this problem, and the approach to measurement should be grounded as much as possible in the drinking behaviour of the study population. Notably, clinical trials registries (e.g., clinicaltrials.gov), CONSORT (16), and some journals, often require specification of the "primary outcome timepoint." A common compromise approach is to measure short term outcomes (1-3 months), medium-term effects (6-9 months), and longer-term outcomes (12-24 months), and to specify the most clinically relevant and realistic of these as primary.

Treatment research has traditionally relied on self-report measures for diagnosis and assessment of treatment outcome, and a number of studies support the validity of this approach under a range of conditions (17,18). There are, however, circumstances in which self-report is inaccurate when compared with a biological measure, such as a breath alcohol test (19).

Where the aim of research is to measure the effects of treatment on habitual heavy alcohol consumption, bio-markers, such as gamma-glutamyl transferase (GGT) or carbohydrate-deficient transferrin (CDT), may be an option. Unfortunately, bio-markers are unsuitable in many target groups, whose use is characterised by intermittent drinking to intoxication rather than chronic heavy drinking; the bio-markers only pick up the latter, and even then, less reliably than self-report with collateral interview (20). Cost is another obstacle–a CDT test costs upwards of US$40 for non-profit research purposes and considerably more for clinical use–with the numbers required for SBI trials making the use of bio-markers an expensive proposition. In addition, the brevity of the opportunity for contact at the point of recruitment makes the collection of blood impracticable in many settings in which SBI is studied. Accordingly, SBI research efforts have to create conditions which maximise the validity of self-report.

Social desirability bias (21) presents arguably the greatest threat to the validity of self report, and it may help explain at least some of the effects attributed to brief intervention. Social desirability bias occurs when study participants under-report socially stigmatised behaviours or over-report socially desirable ones. The problem of social desirability bias has been alleviated with the use of bio-markers in some studies (20,22). In such trials, outcomes measured by self-report and bio-markers were judged to be equivalent, but it is possible that participants who knew their drinking was subject to blood test were less inclined to underreport than they might otherwise have been.

While change in alcohol consumption is typically a primary outcome measure, the goal of intervention is to reduce personal and social costs of unhealthy alcohol use, including illness, injury, reduced quality of life, mortality, and health service expenditure. Most SBI trials include measures from one or more of these domains, often relying solely on self-report, but sometimes utilising administrative data, e.g., emergency department admissions (23) and hospitalisation (24). Curiously, some studies find effects of SBI on consumption and not on problems (25,26), while others find the converse (27).

Minimising the exposure of controls to assessment. The foregoing highlights a challenge in the design and interpretation of treatment studies, and in particular, controlled trials of SBI, namely, the need to maximise the experimental contrast while retaining sufficient baseline assessment to permit appropriate statistical control (28). The problem is that the assessment procedure required to measure consumption and problems at baseline and follow-up is similar in form and content to elements of the intervention being studied, i.e., the provision of motivational feedback requires assessment of the patient's drinking. Accordingly, controls are exposed to part of the intervention. Possible approaches to attenuate this risk include the recruitment of samples of sufficient size to permit assessment of only a portion (a random sample) of each experimental arm at any given follow-up point. A second approach would be to use briefer assessment. Given the emerging evidence supporting briefer forms of screening instruments, e.g., the 3-item AUDIT-C (29), there might be benefit in considering their use in clinical trials to help minimise assessment effects. There may also be value in attempting to measure the tendency toward socially desirable response and to control for it using statistical adjustment of effect estimates, however, the literature remains equivocal on the validity of existing social desirability measures (30). Further research is needed to develop a brief, valid measure of the tendency to giving a socially desirable response, which could be used in SBI trials. Given the paucity of research in this area, there may also be value in conducting a study to determine the effect of screening and assessment, versus screening alone, versus no contact, a placebo contact, or delayed screening.

Other approaches to measuring treatment outcomes include examining health outcomes in administrative data sources, e.g., emergency department utilization, hospital inpatient stays for injury, drink-driving offence data, and traffic crash outcomes. These approaches typically require obtaining patient consent to access these records via data linkage, and the co-operation of the agencies that collect these data. Careful consideration needs to be given to a range of biases attendant in the use of administrative datasets (31,32), which are beyond the scope of this paper.

INTERNAL VERSUS EXTERNAL VALIDITY

The internal validity of a clinical trial is the extent to which systematic error is controlled for in the design and execution of the trial (33). In other words, findings may be considered internally valid to the extent that the investigation permits alternative explanations for observed differences between treatment groups to be ruled out. Central to internal validity of a RCT is appropriate randomisation of participants, ensuring that the intervention is delivered according to protocol, minimising the risk of exposing control participants to the intervention (i.e., contamination), having a sufficiently large study sample to allow the detection of meaningful effects, conducting suitable statistical analyses, and appropriate interpretation of the results (34).

External validity is the extent to which the findings of a trial (with high internal validity) can be generalised to the study population and to conditions of feasible healthcare delivery (33). Studies with highly self-selected study samples, even if bias is minimised, are unlikely to generalise well. This is arguably a weakness of SBI research, in which some treatment protocols cannot be sustainably implemented in practice.

In some situations it may be desirable to trade off some experimental control, and therefore risk a decrement in internal validity, to make gains in external validity. For example, conducting a trial of SBI in a captive audience, such as a class of psychology undergraduates, might assist in keeping attrition low, but the findings would have little relevance to healthcare delivery. Conducting the trial in a primary healthcare setting would make the job of follow-up assessment more difficult, and thereby increase attrition, but the results would generalise better to the kind of setting in which such an intervention could be implemented sustainably.

A related consideration is the extent of the intervention, including how complex it is, and the training required to implement it. More complex interventions requiring higher staff skill levels are more difficult to disseminate. With regard to the growing literature on computerised interventions, consideration should be given to users' access to equipment and technical support. The results of trials of complex or otherwise intensive interventions should be interpreted in terms of the potential for the procedure to become a feature of routine healthcare delivery.

Readiness to change and treatment seeking. Assessing a person's readiness to change is commonly recommended as part of SBI, though it should be noted that measuring readiness–and some argue the construct itself (35)–is problematic, there being little correlation with treatment outcome. In a recent study examining readiness to change, including intentions to abstain or cut-down, only confidence (i.e., self-efficacy) and intention to abstain were associated with drinking six months later (36).

Treatment seeking is closely related to intention to change. In a retrospective analysis of a nationally representative sample in the USA, (37) help seeking was shown to increase the likelihood of recovery from alcohol dependence. The extent to which patient groups in research studies are seeking treatment, have high self-efficacy, and intend to modify their drinking, theoretically affects the external validity of research findings, i.e., studies conducted in highly motivated and capable groups should not be generalised to all persons with unhealthy drinking. It is therefore important that authors specify whether SBI is being tested in people seeking treatment, and it may help to measure self-efficacy and intention to change at baseline. When interpreting the research literature, studies of persons identified via opportunistic screening (i.e., among non-treatment seekers) should be considered separately from those involving persons seeking help, as in the meta-analysis by Moyer et al. (5).

ANALYTICAL ISSUES

Interpreting trial results. Reductions in drinking and/or alcohol-related harm are often observed to varying degree in both intervention and control groups in clinical trials. In a number of published studies, such results have been interpreted as evidence of an intervention effect (38,39). This is problematic for two reasons. First and foremost is regression to the mean, a statistical artefact produced by asymmetric sampling from a population (e.g., via screening), and measurement error (40). In the case of SBI, individuals identified on the basis of their alcohol risk are likely, on average, to report lower levels of consumption and fewer problems when assessed later, in the absence of intervention. The extent of regression to the mean increases in accordance with the risk threshold for receiving intervention (i.e., the higher the screening cut off score), and as the reliability of measures decreases. In studies without a control group, or where reductions occur equally in the intervention and control groups, reductions in the intervention group's drinking cannot reasonably be interpreted as evidence that the intervention was effective.

A second alternative explanation for reductions in drinking in intervention trials is seasonal or other cyclical variation in drinking, and the effect of one-off secular events. Some populations, e.g., college students, exhibit a distinct cyclical rhythm in their drinking behaviour, increasing consumption early in the term and around certain events and holidays, and reducing it before and during examinations. If follow-up assessments are conducted at a time of year when students are less inclined to drinking, within-group comparisons would potentially lead to the erroneous conclusion that the intervention was responsible for behaviour change.

The best means of avoiding an incorrect inference is to randomly assign individuals to an intervention or control group, to assess both groups at the same point in time (i.e., a parallel trial) and to resist the temptation of interpreting within-group change, relying solely on between group comparisons with control for individual measures at baseline (discussed below). Thus, the effects of regression to the mean, seasonality, and unforseen influences, are approximately equally distributed across the groups.

Control for baseline differences. Analysis of trial data should include adjustment of each individual's outcome count/score for their baseline count/score (28). This has two advantages: (1) it controls for differences between the study groups at baseline, thereby reducing the likelihood that these contribute to apparent treatment effects, and (2) it generally increases statistical power to detect treatment effects (28).

Distributional assumptions. When the outcome being modelled is a difference or change–and the difference in means (from baseline or between groups) is often linear (or linear enough)–linear regression is appropriate, and simplest for readers to interpret. Often, however, the outcomes used to assess the efficacy of SBI are based on counts, e.g., the number of drinking days in a specified period, and the typical number of drinks consumed per occasion. The data are not continuous and analysis should therefore be based on distributions for discrete data, such as the Poisson distribution, which has one parameter, meaning that the variance is equal to the mean. An alternative is the negative binomial distribution, which has extra parameters, allowing the variance to be greater than the mean, a feature described as over-dispersion (41). Variants on these models include zero-inflated Poisson and zero-inflated negative binomial, which are discussed in detail elsewhere (42,43). Sometimes it is appropriate to avoid distributional assumptions by dichotomizing the data, and using tests of proportions or logistic regression, e.g., for hazardous drinking status at follow-up: yes versus no.

Recent research examining a range of count models for drinking outcomes in a clinical trial showing null results of SBI for inpatients with unhealthy alcohol use (44), demonstrated that standard Poisson models poorly characterised the alcohol consumption data. Importantly, the probability of Type I error using a Poisson model to compare the randomized groups was remarkably large (23-58%) when the true distribution was an over-dispersed Poisson (42). Given the usual distribution of alcohol consumption data, in which there are numerous zeros (representing abstinence) and some extreme values for very heavy drinking, negative binomial regression is likely to protect against the risk of Type I error (42).

Intention to treat versus treatment received analyses. The appropriate method of analysis for clinical trials data remains a hotly debated topic, principally because of problems created by missing data, compounded by the use of multiple follow-up assessments (45,46). In an intention to treat (ITT) analysis, subjects are analysed in the groups to which they were randomized. The alternative to ITT is a treatment received analysis, which might be useful if many people assigned to brief intervention do not receive it. This can happen in large screening programs in which patients do not proceed to the next step. The obvious limitation of a treatment received analysis is that randomized groups are not being compared, but rather, a subset of those randomized to intervention, which may introduce bias. ITT is the preferred approach because it "gives a pragmatic estimate of the benefit of a change in treatment policy rather than of potential benefit in patients who receive treatment exactly as planned" (47, p. 670). A treatment received analysis can be informative where pragmatic considerations require it, but results should be interpreted with caution.

Missing data. There are various options available for the analysis of trial data in which there are missing values: analysis of only those cases with complete data, use of a modelling approach, as well as various methods based on imputation of missing values. Analysis of only those cases with complete data rests on the assumption that follow-up data are missing at random. It is usually difficult to establish the validity of this assumption, however, quite often, the pattern of loss-to-follow-up suggests that the missing data are unlikely to be systematically related to features of the intervention. For example, in a recent study of web-based SBI in primary healthcare (48), with follow-up assessments six weeks and six months after intervention, approximately equal numbers of participants were lost from each group, with < 5% of cases lacking assessments for both follow-up periods. Those lost to follow-up did not have higher baseline drinking levels than those who remained in the trial.

There are alternatives to excluding cases with missing data, generally based on some form of imputation. Nich and Carroll present a case for a modelling-based method that can account for missing data, namely, the use of random-effects regression (49). In contrast to traditional analytical methods, such as ANOVA, random-effects models allow for use of all the follow-up data, by estimating parameters for each study participant with the available data for that individual and data from the entire sample (50). This approach does not rely on imputation of missing values.

Imputation-based approaches were developed in order account for potential biases arising from participant drop-out in clinical trials (51). Such attrition is often due to unpleasant side-effects of treatment. Excluding such cases from the analysis tends to exaggerate the effectiveness of the treatment. In SBI trials it is uncommon for individuals who consent to participate not to complete the treatment. The challenge is to account for potential biases arising from loss-to-follow-up, rather than failure to complete the intervention.

Common imputation methods for missing follow-up data include filling-forward: replacing a participant's missing follow-up data with a value from an earlier complete follow-up (also known as "last value carried forward"), and filling-back: replacing missing follow-up data with a value from a later follow-up. Such simple imputation has been strongly criticised because it requires very strong assumptions, that behaviour at one point is maintained at the next, thereby "... reduc[ing] error variance, artificially increase[ing] degrees of freedom, and thus increase[ing] the risk of Type I error" (50). The preferred imputation approach is the use of maximum likelihood estimation (52).

REPORTING OF FINDINGS

A multi-disciplinary field. Given the cross-cutting health and social effects of unhealthy alcohol use and the multi-disciplinary nature of research on this problem, the SBI literature reflects a diversity of clinical and academic traditions, including medicine, clinical psychology, nursing, health promotion, and social marketing. Probably as a consequence, the research literature is dispersed across a broad array of journals, which vary considerably in their style, reporting requirements, statistical traditions, and standards of review. It is only recently that the leading medical journals have adopted formal guidelines for the reporting of clinical trials (16); similar guidelines are yet to be implemented for other journals.

The Consolidated Standards of Reporting Trials (CONSORT) statement. The appropriate implementation and reporting of RCTs has received a great deal of attention in the last decade or so (34). The CONSORT guidelines (16,53) consist of a flow diagram demonstrating the passage of study participants through the trial, and a 22-item checklist of information to include in the report (Table 1). Ensuring that the implementation of the trial and the presentation of findings fulfil the CONSORT criteria, is a requirement of several journals, but, irrespective of the journal requirements, complying with the CONSORT is likely to produce a study of high quality and is therefore recommended. The CONSORT checklist is presented in the table below (53).

CHALLENGES IN STUDYING SBI DELIVERED VIA COMPUTERS

There is growing interest in the use of computerised interventions for alcohol problems. This is partly due to the scarcity of time for alcohol interventions within primary care settings. Computerised approaches may help overcome some patients' reluctance to discuss their alcohol consumption, they can assist in ensuring

TABLE 1. CONSORT Checklist of Items to Include When Reporting a Randomized Trial

PAPER SECTION and topic	Item	Description
TITLE & ABSTRACT	1	How participants were allocated to interventions (e.g., "random allocation," "randomized," or "randomly assigned").
INTRODUCTION Background	2	Scientific background and explanation of rationale.
METHODS Participants	3	Eligibility criteria for participants and the settings and locations where the data were collected.
Interventions	4	Precise details of the interventions intended for each group and how and when they were actually administered.
Objectives	5	Specific objectives and hypotheses.
Outcomes	6	Clearly defined primary and secondary outcome measures and, when applicable, any methods used to enhance the quality of measurements (e.g., multiple observations, training of assessors).
Sample size	7	How sample size was determined and, when applicable, explanation of any interim analyses and stopping rules.
Randomization – Sequence generation	8	Method used to generate the random allocation sequence, including details of any restrictions (e.g., blocking, stratification)
Randomization – Allocation concealment	9	Method used to implement the random allocation sequence (e.g., numbered containers or central telephone), clarifying whether the sequence was concealed until interventions were assigned.
Randomization – Implementation	10	Who generated the allocation sequence, who enrolled participants, and who assigned participants to their groups.
Blinding (masking)	11	Whether or not participants, those administering the interventions, and those assessing the outcomes were blinded to group assignment. When relevant, how the success of blinding was evaluated.
Statistical methods	12	Statistical methods used to compare groups for primary outcome(s); Methods for additional analyses, such as subgroup analyses and adjusted analyses.
RESULTS Participant flow	13	Flow of participants through each stage (a diagram is strongly recommended). Specifically, for each group report the numbers of participants randomly assigned, receiving intended treatment, completing the study protocol, and analyzed for the primary outcome. Describe protocol deviations from study as planned, together with reasons.
Recruitment	14	Dates defining the periods of recruitment and follow-up.
Baseline data	15	Baseline demographic and clinical characteristics of each group.
Numbers analyzed	16	Number of participants (denominator) in each group included in each analysis and whether the analysis was by "intention-to-treat". State the results in absolute numbers when feasible (e.g., 10/20, not 50%).
Outcomes and estimation	17	For each primary and secondary outcome, a summary of results for each group, and the estimated effect size and its precision (e.g., 95% confidence interval).
Ancillary analyses	18	Address multiplicity by reporting any other analyses performed, including subgroup analyses and adjusted analyses, indicating those pre-specified and those exploratory.
Adverse events	19	All important adverse events or side effects in each intervention group.
DISCUSSION Interpretation	20	Interpretation of the results, taking into account study hypotheses, sources of potential bias or imprecision and the dangers associated with multiplicity of analyses and outcomes.
Generalizability	21	Generalizability (external validity) of the trial findings.
Overall evidence	22	General interpretation of the results in the context of current evidence.

consistent delivery of interventions, and they can improve access to preventive healthcare. There is potential for employment of these technologies more widely and extending the reach of interventions to people with undiagnosed or untreated alcohol use disorders. A recent study suggests that current drinkers have good internet access (54) and there is considerable support among drinkers for Internet-based interventions (55,56).

Three recent review studies (57-59) confirm the high level of interest among potential users but conclude that there is still insufficient evidence to support their efficacy in reducing unhealthy alcohol use. The few studies employing the RCT design were conducted in healthcare settings, where patients completed the computerised intervention after face-to-face contact with research staff, even if follow-up was accomplished via remote communication. There

TABLE 2. Methodological Problems in Randomized Controlled Trials of SBI and Suggested Solutions

Problem	Solution
Insufficient statistical power	Recruit larger samples Maximise experimental contrast Control for baseline individual scores/counts in analysis
Publication bias	Consult meta-analyses of trials with and without the smaller or lesser quality studies
Assessment effects	Minimise assessment of controls (e.g., using AUDIT-C) Include an unassessed control group or a group with delayed assessment Blind participants to the aims of the study Recruit a large enough initial sample to allow assessment of random sub-samples at follow-up time points Consider using bio-markers for population groups with chronic heavy drinking
Social desirability bias	Use non-judgemental language and assurances of confidentiality Use objective measures, e.g., hospitalisation. Measure participants' tendencies to give socially desirable responses and adjust treatment effects statistically
Poor generalisability of findings to healthcare delivery	Minimise the complexity of the intervention and ensure it could be implemented as part of routine service Conduct the trial in conditions as near to actual service conditions as possible Measure and report whether participants are seeking treatment, their self-efficacy, and intentions to change
Misinterpretation of trial outcomes	Avoid interpreting within-group changes, instead examining between group differences at follow-up, with control for individual counts/scores at baseline Note the recommendations of the CONSORT statement
Invalid statistical arguments	Use analytic methods with valid distributional assumptions Use an *intention to treat* analysis whenever feasible Interpret *treatment received* analyses cautiously Use random effects models to avoid imputation of missing data Avoid simple imputation methods for handling missing data
Poor reporting	Observe the recommendations of the CONSORT statement

are significant challenges in maintaining a sample recruited via the Internet (60,61), and to date, there have been no RCTs published on this intervention approach.

CONCLUSIONS

The primary methodological issues identified in this paper were the need to conduct studies with samples of sufficient size to detect the modest effects expected of SBI, and the importance of designing baseline and follow-up protocols which minimise assessment effects (Table 2). Also discussed was the impracticability of using bio-markers, and the idea of measuring and controlling for the hypothetical effects of social desirability bias and poor recall when measuring treatment outcome, or at least creating conditions for maximum validity of self-report (e.g., by informing subjects they will be tested or assuring anonymity/confidentiality). Greater attention should be given to the generalizability of trial outcomes at the design stage, and therefore to the trade-off between internal and external validity. Analytical issues include the pitfall of interpreting within-group changes, and the importance of randomisation to protect against the effects of regression to the mean and seasonal changes in drinking. Control for baseline differences in post intervention between-group comparisons, the employment of appropriate distributional assumptions in regression analysis, and the treatment of missing data were each examined. Even though it is not a requirement of all of the journals in which SBI trials are reported, authors should consider using the CONSORT statement as a guide to trial design, implementation, and reporting. Given the strong demand for Internet-based interventions, and the feasibility of providing these as a means of addressing unhealthy alcohol use in persons who otherwise do not come to the attention of clinical services, the challenge of designing trials to evaluate these interventions has to be addressed.

REFERENCES

1. Saunders JB, Aasland OG, Babor TF, de la Fuente JR, Grant M. Development of the Alcohol Use Disorders Identification Test (AUDIT): World Health Organisation Collaborative Project on Early Detection of Persons with Harmful Alcohol Consumption–II. Addiction 1993;88(6):791-804.

2. Miller WR, Rollnick S. Motivational interviewing: preparing people to change addictive behavior. New York: Guilford Press; 1991.

3. Saunders JB, Lee NK. Hazardous alcohol use: Its delineation as a subthreshold disorder, and approaches to its diagnosis and management. Comprehensive Psychiatry 2000;41(2 Suppl. 1):95-103.

4. Bertholet N, Daeppen JB, Wietlisbach V, Fleming M, Burnand B. Reduction of alcohol consumption by brief alcohol intervention in primary care: systematic review and meta-analysis. Arch Intern Med 2005; 165(9):986-95.

5. Moyer A, Finney JW, Swearingen CE, Vergun P. Brief interventions for alcohol problems: A meta-analytic review of controlled investigations in treatment-seeking and non-treatment-seeking populations. Addiction 2002;97(3):279-92.

6. US Preventive Services Task Force. Screening and behavioral counseling interventions in primary care to reduce alcohol misuse: recommendation statement. Ann Intern Med 2004;140(7):554-6.

7. Beich A, Gannik D, Malterud K. Screening and brief intervention for excessive alcohol use: qualitative interview study of the experiences of general practitioners. BMJ 2002;325(7369):870.

8. Lock CA, Kaner EF, Heather N, Gilvarry E, McAvoy BR. Changes in receptionists' attitudes towards involvement in a general practice-based trial of screening and brief alcohol intervention. Br J Gen Pract 2000;50(451):111-5.

9. Wright JT, Jr., Dunn JK, Cutler JA, Davis BR, Cushman WC, Ford CE, et al. Outcomes in hypertensive black and nonblack patients treated with chlorthalidone, amlodipine, and lisinopril. JAMA 2005;293(13): 1595-608.

10. Dickersin K. The existence of publication bias and risk factors for its occurrence. JAMA 1990;263(10): 1385-9.

11. Dickersin K, Chan S, Chalmers TC, Sacks HS, Smith H, Jr. Publication bias and clinical trials. Control Clin Trials 1987;8(4):343-53.

12. Jonson H, Hermansson U, Ronnberg S, Gyllenhammar C, Forsberg L. Comments on brief intervention of alcohol problems: a review of a review. Addiction 1995;90(8):1118-21.

13. Bien TH, Miller WR, Tonigan JS. Brief intervention: a reply to a review of a review. Addiction 1995;90:1118-20.

14. Clifford PR, Maisto SA. Subject reactivity effects and alcohol treatment outcome research. J Stud Alcohol 2000;61(6):787-93.

15. Kypri K, Langley JD, Saunders JB, Cashell-Smith ML. Assessment may conceal therapeutic benefit: findings from a randomized controlled trial for hazardous drinking. Addiction 2007;102(1):62-70.

16. Begg C, Cho M, Eastwood S, Horton R, Moher D, Olkin I, et al. Improving the quality of reporting of randomized controlled trials. The CONSORT statement. JAMA 1996;276(8):637-9.

17. Winters KC, Stinchfield RD, Henly GA. Further validation of new scales measuring adolescent alcohol and other drug abuse. Journal of Studies on Alcohol 1993;54(5):534-41.

18. Barnea Z, Rahav G, Teichman M. The reliability and consistency of self-reports on substance use in a longitudinal study. British Journal of Addiction 1987; 82(8):891-8.

19. Midanik L. Over-reports of recent alcohol consumption in a clinical population: a validity study. Drug Alcohol Depend 1982;9(2):101-10.

20. Babor TF, Steinberg K, Anton R, Del Boca F. Talk is cheap: Measuring drinking outcomes in clinical trials. Journal of Studies on Alcohol 2000;61(1):55-63.

21. Crowne DP, Marlowe D. A new scale of social desirability independent of psychopathology. Journal of Consulting Psychology 1960;24:349-354.

22. Anderson P, Scott E. The effect of general practitioners' advice to heavy drinking men. Br J Addict 1992;87(6):891-900.

23. Gentilello LM, Rivara FP, Donovan DM, Jurkovich GJ, Daranciang E, Dunn CW, et al. Alcohol interventions in a trauma center as a means of reducing the risk of injury recurrence. Ann Surg 1999;230(4): 473-80; discussion 480-3.

24. Fleming MF, Barry KL, Manwell LB, Johnson K, London R. Brief physician advice for problem alcohol drinkers. A randomized controlled trial in community-based primary care practices. JAMA 1997;277(13): 1039-45.

25. World Health Organisation Brief Intervention Study Group. A cross-national trial of brief interventions with heavy drinkers. American Journal of Public Health 1996;86(7):948-55.

26. Senft RA, Polen MR, Freeborn DK, Hollis JF. Brief intervention in a primary care setting for hazardous drinkers. American Journal of Preventative Medicine 1997;13(6):464-70.

27. Richmond R, Heather N, Wodak A, Kehoe L, Webster I. Controlled evaluation of a general practice-based brief intervention for excessive drinking. Addiction 1995;90(1):119-32.

28. Vickers AJ, Altman DG. Statistics notes: Analysing controlled trials with baseline and follow up measurements. British Medical Journal 2001;323(7321): 1123-4.

29. Dawson DA, Grant BF, Stinson FS, Zhou Y. Effectiveness of the derived Alcohol Use Disorders Identification Test (AUDIT-C) in screening for alcohol use disorders and risk drinking in the US general population. Alcohol Clin Exp Res 2005;29(5):844-54.

30. Barger SD. The Marlowe-Crowne affair: short forms, psychometric structure, and social desirability. J Pers Assess 2002;79(2):286-305.

31. Langley J, Stephenson S, Cryer C, Borman B. Traps for the unwary in estimating person based injury incidence using hospital discharge data. Inj Prev 2002;8(4):332-7.

32. Stephenson S, Langley J, Cryer C. Effects of service delivery versus changes in incidence on trends in injury: a demonstration using hospitalised traumatic brain injury. Accid Anal Prev 2005;37(5):825-32.

33. Juni P, Altman DG, Egger M. Systematic reviews in health care: Assessing the quality of controlled clinical trials. BMJ 2001;323(7303):42-6.

34. Jadad AR. Randomised controlled trials: a user's guide. London: BMJ Books 1998; 1998.

35. Sutton S. Back to the drawing board? A review of applications of the transtheoretical model to substance use. Addiction 2001;96(1):175-86.

36. Williams E, Horton N, Samet J, Saitz R. Do brief measures of readiness to change predict alcohol consumption and consequences in primary care patients with unhealthy alcohol use? Alcohol Clin Exp Res 2007;31(3):428-35.

37. Dawson D, Grant BF, Stinson FS, Chou PS. Estimating the effect of help-seeking on achieving recovery from alcohol dependence. Addiction 2006;101(6): 824-34.

38. Hester RK, Delaney HD. Behavioral Self-Control Program for Windows: results of a controlled clinical trial. Journal of Consulting and Clinical Psychology 1997;65(4):686-93.

39. Forsberg L, Ekman S, Halldin J, Ronnberg S. Brief interventions for risk consumption of alcohol at an emergency surgical ward. Addictive Behaviors 2000; 25(3):471-5.

40. Morton V, Torgerson DJ. Effect of regression to the mean on decision making in health care. BMJ 2003;326(7398):1083-4.

41. Dean CB. Overdispersion. In: P. Armitage TC, editor. Encyclopedia of Biostatistics. Chichester: J. Wiley & Sons; 1998. Pp. 3226-32.

42. Horton NJ, Kim E, Saitz R. A cautionary note regarding count models of alcohol consumption in randomized controlled trials. BMC Medical Research Methodology 2007;7(9).

43. Horton NJ, Samet JH, Saitz R. Regression methods for counts to model alcohol consumption outcomes. Alcoholism Clinical and Experimental Research 2004; 28(Suppl):165.

44. Saitz R, Palfai TP, Cheng DM, Horton NJ, Freedmer N, Dukes K, et al. Brief intervention for medical inpatients with unhealthy alcohol use: a randomized, controlled trial. Annals of Interal Medicine 2007;146: 167-76.

45. Howard KI, Krause MS, Orlinsky DE. The attrition dilemma: toward a new strategy for psychotherapy research. J Consult Clin Psychol 1986;54(1):106-10.

46. Nich C, Carroll K. Now you see it, now you don't: a comparison of traditional versus random-effects regression models in the analysis of longitudinal follow-up data from a clinical trial. J Consult Clin Psychol 1997;65(2):252-61.

47. Hollis S, Campbell F. What is meant by intention to treat analysis? Survey of published randomised controlled trials. BMJ 1999;319:670-4.

48. Kypri K, Saunders JB, Williams SM, McGee RO, Langley JD, Cashell-Smith ML, et al. Web-based screening and brief intervention for hazardous drinking: a double-blind randomised controlled trial. Addiction 2004;99(11):1410-7.

49. Laird NM, Ware JH. Random-effects models for longitudinal data. Biometrics 1982;38(4):963-74.

50. Nich C, Carroll K. Now you see it, now you don't: a comparison of traditional versus random-effects regression models in the analysis of longitudinal follow-up data from a clinical trial. Journal of Consulting and Clinical Psychology 1997;65(2):252-61.

51. Nich C, Carroll KM. 'Intention to treat' meets 'missing data': Implications of alternate strategies for analyzing clinical trials data. Drug & Alcohol Dependence 2002;68(2) Oct 2002:US http://www.

52. Gorbein JA, Lazaro CG, Little RJA. Incomplete data in repeated measures analysis. Statistical Methods in Medical Research 1992;1:275-95.

53. Moher D, Schulz KF, Altman D. CONSORT Checklist of items to include when reporting a randomized trial, http://www.consort-statement.org/Statement/revisedstatement.htm, accessed 30 December 2006. In: 2001.

54. Cunningham JA, Selby PL, Kypri K, Humphreys KN. Access to the Internet among drinkers, smokers and illicit drug users: is it a barrier to the provision of interventions on the World Wide Web? Med Inform Internet Med 2006;31(1):53-8.

55. Saitz R, Helmuth ED, Aromaa SE, Guard A, Belanger M, Rosenbloom DL. Web-based screening and brief intervention for the spectrum of alcohol problems. Prev Med 2004;39(5):969-75.

56. Kypri K, Saunders JB, Gallagher SJ. Acceptability of various brief intervention approaches for hazardous drinking among university students. Alcohol and Alcoholism 2003;38(6):626-8.

57. Copeland J, Martin G. Web-based interventions for substance use disorders: a qualitative review. J Subst Abuse Treat 2004;26(2):109-16.

58. Kypri K, Sitharthan T, Cunningham JA, Kavanagh DJ, Dean JI. Innovative approaches to intervention for problem drinking. Current Opinion in Psychiatry 2005; 18(3):229-34.

59. Finfgeld-Connett D. Web-based treatment for problem drinking. J Psychosoc Nurs Ment Health Serv 2006;44(9):20-7.

60. Linke S, Brown A, Wallace P. Down your drink: a web-based intervention for people with excessive alcohol consumption. Alcohol Alcohol 2004;39(1):29-32.

61. Cunningham JA, Humphreys K, Koski-Jannes A. Providing personalized assessment feedback for problem drinking on the Internet: A pilot project. Journal of Studies on Alcohol 2000;61(6):794-8.

doi:10.1300/J465v28n03_04

Communication During Brief Intervention, Intention to Change, and Outcome

Jean-Bernard Daeppen, MD
Nicolas Bertholet, MD
Gerhard Gmel, PhD
Jacques Gaume, MA

SUMMARY. *Objectives*: To explore the relationship between patient's intention to change regarding future alcohol consumption following brief alcohol intervention (BAI) and changes in alcohol consumption 12-months later and the communication characteristics between patient and counselor during BAI.

Design, Setting and Subjects: Data from 367 patients (experimental arm) of a pragmatic randomized controlled trial were used to assess the effectiveness of BAI among hazardous drinkers attending an Emergency Department (Lausanne University Hospital, Lausanne, Switzerland). Alcohol outcome measures at baseline and 12 months follow-up included usual number of drinks per week, monthly frequency of heavy episodic drinking (5 or more standard drinks for men; 4 or more for women), and the Alcohol Use Disorders Identification Test (AUDIT) score. In addition, the communication characteristics between patient and counselor were analyzed via tape recordings using the Motivational Interviewing Skill Code (MISC) from 97 participants. Patient readiness and importance to change on a 10-point Likert scale (readiness/importance to change ruler) was asked during BAI, and patient intention to change alcohol consumption (yes/no) was asked at the last step. Differences in alcohol outcome at follow-up between the 367 patients who did or did not have an intention to change consumption at baseline were compared, as were differences between these two groups in communication characteristics for the 97 who completed tape recordings.

Results: Patients with an intention to decrease alcohol consumption reduced alcohol use and related problems more often, and reported higher levels of importance and readiness to change than did their counterparts. Analyses of MISC-coded data showed a significantly higher use of MI-consistent skills among those with a moderation intention, but no group differences on the 8 other counselor communication skills measures were found. Analyses of patient speech during the intervention indicated that those with an intention to change their alcohol consumption significantly more often self-explored personal ambivalence towards alcohol, expressed more intensely their ability, commitment, desire, need and reason to change their alcohol use than did those in the no decrease group.

Conclusions: The intention expressed by hazardous drinkers when concluding BAI is associated with both patient change talk during BAI and drinking outcome 12 months later, but is mainly

---

Jean-Bernard Daeppen, Gerhard Gmel, and Jacques Gaume are affiliated with the Alcohol Treatment Center, Department of Community Medicine and Health, Lausanne University Hospital, Lausanne, Switzerland.

Nicolas Bertholet is affiliated with the Clinical Addiction Research and Education (CARE) Unit, Section of General Internal Medicine, Boston Medical Center and Boston University School of Medicine, Boston, MA, USA.

Address correspondence to: Dr. Jean-Bernard Daeppen, CTA, Mont-Paisible 16, 1011 Lausanne, Switzerland (E-mail: jean-bernard.daeppen@chuv.ch).

[Haworth co-indexing entry note]: "Communication During Brief Intervention, Intention to Change, and Outcome." Daeppen, Jean-Bernard et al. Co-published simultaneously in *Substance Abuse* (The Haworth Medical Press, an imprint of The Haworth Press, Inc.) Vol. 28, No. 3, 2007, pp. 43-51; and: *Alcohol/Drug Screening and Brief Intervention: Advances in Evidence-Based Practice* (ed: Richard Saitz, and Marc Galanter) The Haworth Medical Press, an imprint of The Haworth Press, Inc., 2007, pp. 43-51. Single or multiple copies of this article are available for a fee from The Haworth Document Delivery Service [1-800-HAWORTH, 9:00 a.m. - 5:00 p.m. (EST). E-mail address: docdelivery@haworthpress.com].

Available online at http://suba.haworthpress.com

doi:10.1300/J465v28n03_05

independent of counselor communication skills. This intention may be an important clinical indicator of which hazardous drinkers are most likely to improve after BAI. doi:10.1300/J465v28n03_05 *[Article copies available for a fee from The Haworth Document Delivery Service: 1-800-HAWORTH. E-mail address: <docdelivery@haworthpress.com> Website: <http://www.HaworthPress.com>*

KEYWORDS. Brief alcohol intervention, intention, patient adherence, communication characteristics, motivational interviewing skills code, counselor skills

INTRODUCTION

Several systematic reviews and meta-analyses support the belief that brief alcohol intervention (BAI) is effective in reducing hazardous alcohol use in a variety of patients.[1-5] However, this aggregated effect might help obscure the fact that not all patients gain from BAI. Following BAI, some patients (independently of their drinking patterns) will demonstrate major changes in their alcohol use, stay the same, or even increase drinking. Little is known about the patient or counselor characteristics associated with behavior changes. Several authors have looked at moderators (characteristics) of BAI efficacy that influence the degree to which behavior change occurs, such as patient gender,[1] age,[6,7] severity of alcohol use disorder,[8] counselor empathy and directiveness[3,9] and type of BAI (e.g., duration, number of sessions[3,10]).

Patient readiness to change[11] may also moderate behavior change resulting from BAI. Gains made by some patients might be due to contemplated changes among those who have high levels of readiness to change. Here, even brief exposure may trigger relatively important and long-lasting behavior changes, where for other patient's interventions that are much more intensive may be of little help.[12] One study[13] concluded, after examining the relative value of readiness or underlying motivational dimensions of perceived desire, ability, or reasons to change alcohol or drug use, that commitment was the final common pathway in the process of change. Many patients might have high levels of readiness, but lack firm commitment to change, thus showing poorer drinking outcomes in many of the BAI studies. Since the final step of BAI often incorporates asking patients their intention, those who commit to moderation are probably more likely to actually reduce their alcohol use by follow-up.

BAI generally incorporates motivational interviewing (MI) style and techniques for use in time-limited health care settings.[14-17] In MI-style BAI, characteristics related to patient commitment, expressed by an objective of drinking moderation or abstinence, might influence drinking outcome. The Motivational Interviewing Skill Code (MISC) quantifies communication characteristics and behaviors of counselors and patients through analyses of video or tape recordings[18-20] and includes a measure of the patient's commitment to change. Since BAI works differentially for patients, it seems worthwhile to explore the relationships between the communication characteristics during BAI, the intention at the end of BAI, and the evolution of alcohol use between baseline and follow-up.

This paper has the goal of estimating whether or not an objective of alcohol use reduction set by patients at the end of BAI is associated with actual reduction 12 months later. However, this estimation would not allow many conclusions to be drawn regarding the content of BAI and how it influences patients' intention to change their alcohol consumption. For example, counselors might perform better during BAI if they believe that a patient is ready to change; conversely, a superior performance of counselors could lead to a stronger patient commitment to change by the end of BAI. Thus, a secondary goal is to evaluate the relationship between patients' intention to change and the communication characteristics during BAI using the Motivational Interviewing Skill Code (MISC) on the 97 subjects with taped BAI.

METHODS

Sample

This study was part of a randomized controlled trial in an Emergency Department (ED) aimed at evaluating the efficacy of BAI in decreasing hazardous alcohol consumption during a 12-month follow-up, as described in detail in another paper (Daeppen et al., submitted). Briefly, there were 8,833 patients attending the ED who were screened; of these 1,366 were positive for hazardous alcohol consumption, defined according to NIAAA standards as men under 65 years old who drink more than 14 drinks per week or more than 4 drinks on a single occasion in the past 30 days, and men over 65 years old and women who drink more than 7 drinks per week or more than 3 drinks on a single occasion. One drink was defined as a regular glass of wine, a regular beer, or a single shot spirit, straight or mixed in a soft drink. After signing informed consent, 486 patients were randomized to a BAI group and 880 to two control groups; of these 367 (75.5%) of the BAI patients and 688 (78.2%) of the control patients were successfully followed-up at 12 months. The analyses reported focus on the 367 patients who completed both BAI and the follow-up in order to evaluate the difference in alcohol use from baseline to 12-months later. The local ethics committee approved the entire protocol.

Counselor

Counselors were six masters level psychologists and one experienced nurse, all with a minimum of one year of clinical practice. A senior physician and a psychologist experienced in teaching motivational interviewing and BAI trained the counselors, first with a 2-day workshop on motivational interviewing containing exercises aimed at improving performance using an active, empathic listening style that minimizes confrontation[21] and second with a 5-day workshop focused on trial information procedures as well as on practice of the 6-step standardized BAI. Supervision was ongoing during the project, either in the presence of patients or through tape recordings of the BAI.

Research Procedures

A single 15-minute motivational style BAI consisting of six steps was performed. At the fifth step, counselors asked patients a question about whether or not they felt ready (based on what happened in BAI) to set an objective regarding their drinking. Patients were then dichotomized into either the group who expressed an objective to decrease or quit drinking (N = 134) or the group who did not (N = 233).

Alcohol use was measured by the weekly drinking amount calculated as the number of standard drinks usually consumed per week and by the frequency of heavy drinking measured by the average occurrence of having 5 standard drinks or more on one occasion for males under 65 years old (4 standard drinks or more on one occasion for males over 65 years old and for females) per month over the last 12-months. Patient alcohol consumption was assessed at baseline and at the 12-months follow-up. The AUDIT score was computed at baseline and at twelve months to serve as a measure of severity of alcohol use disorder.[22] The importance and readiness to change at baseline were estimated using a readiness ruler assessing importance and readiness to change on a 1-10 Likert scale, one being "not important at all–not ready at all–to change my drinking now" and 10 being "very important–ready–to change my drinking now."[23] Finally, the counselor subjectively evaluated the effectiveness of BAI immediately after BAI and assigned patients to a group that deemed BAI "rather or very effective" or to another group of "all others."

In order to explore the relationship between patients' intention to change and the communication characteristics during BAI, 166 consecutive BAI sessions were tape-recorded with patient permission and 97 of these were eligible for coding and analyses. Excluded were 33 lost to follow-up, 25 with incomplete records, 7 with mismatched identification codes, 3 who were not sufficiently fluent in French, and 1 whose wife intruded during the session. Two masters level psychologists independently completed the Motivational Interviewing Skills Code (MISC) coding, blinded to data from assessment and follow-up; both were trained in motivational interviewing and in using the MISC, Version 2.0.[19]

The MISC is comprised of global ratings and behavior counts. Two passes were made through each taped session: the first to assess global ratings on 7-point Likert scales and the second to assign behavior counts. For the current analyses, 9 items of counselor talk and 7 items of patient talk were selected for their clinical relevance to BAI. Counselor items were (1) *Acceptance*, (2) *Empathy*, and (3) *MI Spirit* global ratings; (4) frequency of *MI-consistent skills* (*Advise with permission*, *Affirm*, *Emphasize control*, *Open question*, *Simple* and *Complex Reflections*, and *Support*); (5) frequency of *MI-inconsistent skills* (i.e., the addition of the behavior counts *Advise without permission*, *Confront*, *Direct*, *Raise concern without permission*, and *Warn*); (6) *MI-consistent skills percentage* as the proportion of the sum of MI-consistent skills and MI-inconsistent skills; (7) *Reflections/Questions ratio*; (8) *Open questions percentage* as the proportion of the sum of open and closed questions; and (9) *Complex reflections percentage* as the proportion of the sum of complex and simple reflections.[18] Patient items were (1) *Self exploration* global rating and 6 behavior counts expressed as the average strength of inclination measured on a scale from −5 (strong inclination away from change) to + 5 (strong inclination toward change) for 6 kinds of "Change talk": (2) *Ability or inability to change*, (3) *Commitment to change or not to change*, (4) *Desire to change or not to change*, (5) *Need to change versus lack of need for change, or a need not to change*, (6) *Reasons to change or reasons not to change*, and (7) *Taking steps toward or away from change*.

Data Analyses

Socio-demographic characteristics, alcohol use and related characteristics and the selected MISC variables were compared at baseline and at follow-up using Pearson's Chi Square test for categorical variables, and Wilcoxon's nonparametric test for continuous variables since asymmetric distributions and heterogeneity of variances for the two groups were frequently seen.

Intra-class correlation coefficients (ICC) of selected MISC variables between the two coders were high, suggesting fair to excellent inter-rater reliability, as reported elsewhere (Gaume et al., submitted).

RESULTS

Table 1 shows baseline demographics and alcohol consumption data on the 367 hazardous drinkers included in the BAI arm of the study. The sample consists mostly of men in their late thirties, of whom about two-thirds are employed and about one-third have college or equivalent education degrees. Their weekly alcohol use, heavy drinking frequency and AUDIT scores are comparable to profiles of average "low-grade hazardous drinkers" (average 13 drinks per week, 4 heavy drinking occasions per month and an AUDIT score of 9). They had relatively low readiness ruler's scores (importance and readiness to change drinking habits) and counselors considered that BAI would be effective for less than 50% of them.

Table 1 also compares the characteristics of the 97 patients with taped sessions to those of the 270 non-coded BAI patients and lists the relevant statistical outcomes in order to determine if findings could be appropriately generalized to the larger sample. The groups had similar demographic characteristics, alcohol use and AUDIT scores. However, the MISC-coded BAI group was significantly higher on the readiness ruler and showed a trend ($p = .06$) towards higher counselor ratings of probable BAI effectiveness than did the non-coded counterparts.

Table 2 compares patients with or without an intention to decrease their alcohol use and AUDIT scores at baseline and 12-month follow-up, as well as on importance and readiness to change and subjective counselor ratings at baseline. Patients with a decrease objective demonstrated significantly greater reductions in weekly drinking amounts, heavy drinking episodes per month and AUDIT scores from baseline to follow-up than did the no decrease counterparts. They also had significantly higher levels of importance and readiness to change, as well as a higher percentage of counselor ratings of BAI effectiveness.

Table 2 also reveals that the decrease objective group initially drank significantly more and had higher AUDIT scores than those in the

TABLE 1. Socio-Demographic Information and Alcohol Consumption–Comparison Between MISC-Coded and Non-Coded BAI in Hazardous Drinkers with 12-Month Follow-Up (N = 367).

	Total (N=367)	MISC-Coded BAI (N=97)	Non-Coded BAI (N=270)	p
Demographic data				
Age, Mean (SD)	39.3 (17.0)	38.4 (17.1)	39.7 (16.9)	0.42 (w)
Sex, % Male (N)	75.7 (278)	80.4 (78)	74.1 (200)	0.21 (c)
Education, % College degree (N)	35.1 (124)	30.5 (29)	36.8 (95)	0.27 (c)
Occupation, % Employed (N)	61.3 (225)	57.7 (56)	62.6 (169)	0.40 (c)
Weekly drinking amount				
Baseline, Mean (SD)	13.0 (11.4)	13.4 (10.2)	12.8 (11.7)	0.45 (w)
12-month follow-up, Mean (SD)	10.9 (11.8)	11.8 (13.3)	10.5 (11.3)	0.72 (w)
Baseline to follow-up difference, Mean (SD)	2.1 (10.8)	1.5 (11.5)	2.3 (10.5)	0.98 (w)
Heavy drinking episodes per month				
Baseline, Mean (SD)	4.3 (6.6)	4.3 (6.2)	4.4 (6.8)	0.65 (w)
12-month follow-up, Mean (SD)	3.6 (6.0)	4.7 (7.5)	3.3 (5.3)	0.30 (w)
Baseline to follow-up difference, Mean (SD)	0.8 (7.0)	-0.2 (5.6)	1.1 (7.4)	0.18 (w)
AUDIT Score				
Baseline; mean (SD)	9.1 (4.9)	9.5 (4.5)	9.0 (5.0)	0.10 (w)
12-month follow-up, Mean (SD)	7.3 (4.6)	7.4 (4.3)	7.2 (4.7)	0.62 (w)
Baseline to follow-up difference, Mean (SD)	1.8 (4.5)	2.1 (4.5)	1.7 (4.5)	0.20 (w)
Readiness Rulers Scores (baseline)				
Importance [1-10], Mean (SD)	3.7 (2.4)	4.4 (2.5)	3.5 (2.3)	0.01 (w)
Readiness [1-10], Mean (SD)	4.2 (2.8)	4.9 (3.0)	3.9 (2.7)	0.04 (w)
Counselor subjective evaluation of BAI effectiveness (baseline)				
% "rather effective" or "very effective" (N)	44.0 (160)	52.1 (50)	41.0 (110)	0.06 (c)

Note: (c) = Pearson's Chi Square test, (w) = Wilcoxon W test.
MISC : Motivational interviewing skill code
BAI : Brief alcohol intervention

other group. The AUDIT scores of the decrease objective patients, though much lower at follow-up, remained significantly higher than those found in the no decrease patients.

Table 3 examines the communications of counselor and patients during BAI by drinking intention among the 97 taped and MISC-coded patients. Of the nine counselor speech elements, no differences existed between decrease and no decrease patients on 8 of them; the single exception being that counselors used significantly more MI-consistent skills within the decrease group. Of the 7 patient speech elements, all but 2 (ability/inability to change and taking steps toward change) had significantly higher frequencies in the decrease objective group. Here, the patients did more self-exploration of ambivalence towards alcohol and expressed with more intensity their ability, commitment, desire, need and reason to change their drinking, compared to counterparts.

DISCUSSION

Results indicate that an objective of alcohol use reduction set by the patient near the end of BAI is associated with more patient self-exploration and change talk during BAI, higher baseline importance and readiness to change, and reduced alcohol use and problems 12 months later. This suggests that the patient intention to

TABLE 2. Alcohol Use and Other Characteristics According to Patient Intention Immediately Following BAI (N = 367).

	Intention		
	Decrease (N=134)	No decrease (N=233)	p value
Weekly drinking amount			
Baseline, Mean (SD)	15.6 (14.0)	11.5 (9.2)	0.01 (w)
12-month follow-up, Mean (SD)	12.5 (16.1)	9.9 (8.4)	0.97 (w)
Baseline to 12-month difference, Mean (SD)	3.1 (13.3)	1.5 (9.0)	0.02 (w)
Heavy drinking episodes per month			
Baseline, Mean (SD)	6.0 (7.9)	3.4 (5.6)	0.00 (w)
12-month follow-up, Mean (SD)	3.9 (6.4)	3.5 (5.7)	0.83 (w)
Baseline to 12-month difference, Mean (SD)	2.3 (8.4)	-0.1 (6.0)	0.00 (w)
AUDIT Score			
Baseline, Mean (SD)	11.2 (6.1)	7.9 (3.5)	0.00 (w)
12-month follow-up, Mean (SD)	8.3 (6.1)	6.6 (3.4)	0.03 (w)
Baseline to 12-month difference, Mean (SD)	2.8 (5.7)	1.3 (3.5)	0.00 (w)
Readiness Rulers Scores (baseline)			
Importance [1-10], Mean (SD)	5.2 (2.5)	2.9 (1.9)	0.00 (w)
Readiness [1-10], Mean (SD)	5.7 (2.4)	3.2 (2.6)	0.00 (w)
Counselor subjective evaluation of BAI effectiveness (baseline)			
% "rather effective" or "very effective" (N)	71.6 (96)	27.8 (64)	0.00 (c)

Note: (c) = Pearson's Chi Square test, (w) = Wilcoxon W test.

change might be a moderator of BAI effectiveness, perhaps reflecting patient commitment to change, which then predicts favorable alcohol use outcome. Commitment has been known to be a major influence in behavioral change processes.[13] Understanding the development of patient intention (commitment) could help maximize BAI strategies. A few studies have investigated the moderators of effectiveness in BAI trials. In chemical dependence treatment studies,[12] a modest relationship has been found between components of 12-step programs that include commitment to abstinence (which could be considered a particular form of intention to change) and outcome. Other ingredients of MI-style BAI that seem to be useful in behavioral therapy paradigms were an increase of self-efficacy,[25] engagement in the process,[26] and readiness to change.[11]

In the present study, counselor skills and communication characteristics of patients were both expected to be instrumental in changing drinking outcomes. It was surprising that only one of the 9 elements (i.e., MI-consistent skills) was significant. Perhaps counselors tend to be more empathic and motivational when they view a patient as less resistant to the whole process and more willing to change.

These findings suggest that BAI might be modified such that they could increase the proportion of patients who at the end of a BAI have a drinking objective to cut down or quit, i.e., a revision of BAI with a special focus on change talk or a modification in BAI training with the particular aim of providing counselors with MI-consistent skills. An alternative would be a case finding strategy that selects the patients who are more likely to benefit from BAI, for example, those with initial higher level of intention to change.

Interestingly, data reported also indicate that patients who set an objective of alcohol use re-

TABLE 3. Communication Characteristics (MISC) During a Brief Alcohol Intervention According to Patient Intention (N = 97).

		Intention		
		Decrease N=36	No decrease N=61	p (Wilcoxon)
Counselor	Acceptance [1-7]	5.9 (0.7)	5.9 (0.7)	0.91
	Empathy [1-7]	5.5 (0.7)	5.5 (0.7)	0.84
	MI Spirit [1-7]	5.6 (0.7)	5.4 (0.7)	0.31
	MI-consistent skills [Freq]	34.9 (8.9)	30.5 (11.1)	0.01
	MI-inconsistent skills [Freq]	1.2 (1.7)	1.2 (1.4)	0.76
	% MI-consistent skills [a]	96.7 (4.1)	96.3 (4.0)	0.48
	Ratio Reflections/Questions [b]	1.1 (0.5)	1.0 (0.5)	0.59
	% Open questions [c]	51.2 (12.5)	53.6 (13.1)	0.48
	% Complex reflections [d]	45.5 (11.2)	45.8 (13.2)	0.80
Patient	Self-exploration [1-7]	5.5 (0.8)	5.0 (0.7)	0.00
	Ability/inability to change [+5 to -5]	0.8 (1.3)	0.4 (0.9)	0.08
	Commitment to change or not to change [+5 to -5]	1.0 (1.5)	-0.7 (1.6)	0.00
	Desire to change or not to change [+5 to -5]	-1.0 (1.6)	-1.9 (1.0)	0.01
	Need to change / Lack of need to change or a need not to change [+5 to -5]	1.0 (1.2)	-0.8 (1.5)	0.00
	Reasons to change or not to change [+5 to -5]	0.3 (0.6)	-0.5 (0.7)	0.00
	Taking steps toward change / away from change [+5 to -5]	1.2 (1.1)	1.1 (0.9)	0.64

[a] % MI-consistent skills: MI-consistent skills / (MI-consistent skills + MI-inconsistent skills)
[b] Ratio Reflections/Questions: Total reflections / Total questions
[c] % Open questions: Total open questions / Total questions (open + closed)
[d] % Complex reflections: Total complex reflections / Total reflections (complex + simple)
MISC : Motivational interviewing Skill Code

duction consumed more alcohol, had more heavy drinking episodes and higher AUDIT scores at baseline. This suggests that objectives to decrease alcohol use reduction are more likely to occur in individuals having higher levels of alcohol use and problems, while patients with less severe hazardous drinking feel less pressure to set drinking reduction objectives and to change their consumption habits. BAI may be most useful after patients reach a certain threshold of hazardous drinking and are more amenable to seeking and receiving help.

Despite some methodological strengths in this study, such as efforts to maximize the internal validity of BAI used (specification of the theoretical model, i.e., motivational interviewing; uniformity of counselor training and attention to fidelity of interventions during the trial), and high agreement between MISC raters, some limitations to the generalizability of these findings should be acknowledged. Most of the socio-demographic and alcohol consumption data of taped and MISC-coded versus non-coded BAI were similar, yet there were differences in readiness ruler scores and counselor subjective evaluations of the efficacy of BAI. This suggests that somehow the recording process itself modified the course of BAI, perhaps because patients ready to change their drinking would be more likely to accept to be recorded. Sample selectivity arising from counselor choice of patient to record can probably be ruled out, since consecutive patients were asked to do this; in any case, these group differences preclude generalizing findings to the non-coded group. There were a relatively small number (97) of MISC-coded BAI patients; this may present a statistical power problem. The confounding of higher alcohol consumption and greater readiness to change among patients who set decrease objectives makes it difficult to determine which of the two provide the greatest impetus to reduce drinking at follow-up.

Several other potential limitations should be mentioned. The MISC was designed for analyses of MI, not BAI, although common skills and common target (behavior change) of MI and BAI suggest that the MISC might well be used to study BAI content. Using the MISC in French also might be a concern as it is a linguistic coding instrument, developed in English and so far not validated in French. Another limitation might arise due to the nature of ED, where time and medical constraints are quite different than those found in other settings (e.g., primary care), and might lead to specific behaviors and attitudes that unduly influence BAI. Self-selection bias may have been introduced by assessing only patients who were willing to participate and have their data recorded, and to cooperate with a follow-up one year later. Since these findings are in a relatively small sample observed prospectively, it would be helpful to repeat and expand such study to allow use of more complex statistical methods to study mechanisms of behavior change, which is currently a NIAAA priority. Future BAI research should try to probe the interaction effects of higher alcohol consumption/higher readiness to change scores among patients with an intention to reduce alcohol use and identify predictors of BAI effectiveness that could be assessed in advance of any intervention attempts. Even with these caveats, the present preliminary results point to the feasibility of optimizing effectiveness and reducing the costs of BAI in ED settings by focusing on patients who are willing to change.

REFERENCES

1. Bertholet N, Daeppen JB, Wietlisbach V, Fleming M, Burnand B: Reduction of alcohol consumption by brief alcohol intervention in primary care: systematic review and meta-analysis. Arch Intern Med 2005; 165: 986-995.

2. Dunn C, Deroo L, Rivara FP: The use of brief interventions adapted from motivational interviewing across behavioral domains: a systematic review. Addiction 2001; 96: 1725-1742.

3 Bien TH, Miller WR, Tonigan JS: Brief interventions for alcohol problems: a review. Addiction 1993; 88: 315-335.

4 D'Onofrio G, Degutis LC: Preventive care in the emergency department: screening and brief intervention for alcohol problems in the emergency department: a systematic review. Acad Emerg Med 2002; 9: 627-638.

5. Emmen MJ, Schippers GM, Bleijenberg G, Wollersheim H: Effectiveness of opportunistic brief interventions for problem drinking in a general hospital setting: systematic review. BMJ 2004; 328: 318.

6. Grossberg PM, Brown DD, Fleming MF: Brief physician advice for high-risk drinking among young adults. Ann Fam Med 2004; 2: 474-480.

7. Fleming MF, Manwell LB, Barry KL, Adams W, Stauffacher EA: Brief physician advice for alcohol problems in older adults: a randomized community-based trial. J Fam Pract 1999; 48: 378-384.

8 Fleming MF, Barry K, Manwell L, Johnson K, London R: Brief physician advice for problem alcohol drinkers. JAMA 1997; 13: 1039-1045.

9. Karno MP, Longabaugh R: An examination of how therapist directiveness interacts with patient anger and reactance to predict alcohol use. J Stud Alcohol 2005; 66: 825-832.

10. Woolard RH, Carty K, Wirtz P, Longabaugh R, Nirenberg TD, Minugh PA: Research fundamentals: follow-up of subjects in clinical trials: addressing subject attrition. Acad Emerg Med 2004; 11: 859-866.

11. DiClemente CC, Schlundt D, Gemmell L: Readiness and stages of change in addiction treatment. Am J Addict 2004; 13: 103-119.

12. Barnett NP, Lebeau-Craven R, O'Leary TA, Colby SM, Rohsenow DJ, Monti PM: Predictors of motivation to change after medical treatment for drinking-related events in adolescents. Psychol Addict Behav 2002; 16: 106-112.

13. Amrhein PC, Miller WR, Yahne CE, Palmer M, Fulcher L: Client commitment language during motivational interviewing predicts drug use outcomes. J Consult Clin Psychol 2003; 71: 862-878.

14. Noonan WC, Moyers TB: Motivational interviewing: a review. Journal of Substance Misuse 1997; 2: 8-16.

15. Dunn C, Deroo L, Rivara FP: The use of brief interventions adapted from motivational interviewing across behavioral domains: a systematic review. Addiction 2001; 96: 1725-1742.

16. Burke BL, Arkowitz H, Menchola M: The efficacy of motivational interviewing: a meta-analysis of controlled clinical trials. Journal of Consulting & Clinical Psychology 2003; 71: 843-861.

17. Vasilaki EI, Hosier SG, Cox WM: The efficacy of motivational interviewing as a brief intervention for excessive drinking: a meta-analytic review. Alcohol Alcohol 2006; 41: 328-335.

18. Miller WR. Motivational Interviewing Skill Code (MISC) Coder's Manual. http://casaa unm edu/download/misc1 pdf [2000

19. Miller WR, Moyers TB, Ernst D, Amrhein PC: Manual for the Motivational Interviewing Skill Code (MISC) Version 2.0. http://casaa unm edu/download/misc pdf [2003

20. Moyers TB, Miller WR, Hendrickson SM: How does motivational interviewing work? Therapist interpersonal skill predicts client involvement within motivational interviewing sessions. J Consult Clin Psychol 2005; 73: 590-598.

21. Baer JS, Rosengren DB, Dunn CW, Wells EA, Ogle RL, Hartzler B: An evaluation of workshop training in motivational interviewing for addiction and mental health clinicians. Drug Alcohol Depend 2004; 73: 99-106.

22. Allen JP, Litten RZ, Fertig JB, Babor T: A review of research on the Alcohol Use Disorders Identification Test (AUDIT). Alcohol Clin Exp Res 1997; 21: 613-619.

23. Hesse M: The Readiness Ruler as a measure of readiness to change poly-drug use in drug abusers. Harm Reduct J 2006; 3:3.

24. Morgenstern J, Frey RM, McCrady BS, Labouvie E, Neighbors CJ: Examining mediators of change in traditional chemical dependency treatment. J Stud Alcohol 1996; 57(1):53-64.

25. Morgenstern J, Longabaugh R: Cognitive-behavioral treatment for alcohol dependence: a review of evidence for its hypothesized mechanisms of action. Addiction 2000; 95: 1475-1490.

26. Dearing RL, Barrick C, Dermen KH, Walitzer KS: Indicators of client engagement: influences on alcohol treatment satisfaction and outcomes. Psychol Addict Behav 2005; 19: 71-78.

doi:10.1300/J465v28n03_05

Examining Quality Issues in Alcohol Misuse Screening

Eric J. Hawkins, PhD
Daniel R. Kivlahan, PhD
Emily C. Williams, MPH
Steven M. Wright, PhD
Thomas Craig, MD, MPH
Katharine A. Bradley, MD, MPH

SUMMARY. The Veterans Health Administration (VHA) has successfully implemented evidence-based alcohol misuse screening with the AUDIT-C. The purpose of this study was to evaluate clinical alcohol screening during the first year after implementation. Using medical record review and mailed patient surveys collected during 2004 by VHA Office of Quality and Performance, this study analyzed concordance of screening results among patients with AUDIT-Cs in both data sources. Among 1,637 patients with AUDIT-C from both sources within 90 days, the medical record screening prevalence rate of alcohol misuse, 24.6% (95% CI: 22.5% to 26.7%), was significantly lower than the survey rate, 33.4% (31.1% to 35.7%). Of 8,312 patients identified as nondrinkers in medical records, 24% reported past year alcohol use and 5% screened positive for alcohol misuse on surveys. Lower rates of alcohol use and misuse documented in medical records compared to mailed surveys suggest further investigation and standardization of clinical screening are necessary. doi:10.1300/J465v28n03_06 *[Article copies available for a fee from The Haworth Document Delivery Service: 1-800-HAWORTH. E-mail address: <docdelivery@haworthpress.com> Website: <http://www.HaworthPress.com>]*

Eric J. Hawkins and Daniel R. Kivlahan are affiliated with Health Services Research & Development, Center of Excellence in Substance Abuse Treatment and Education, VA Puget Sound Health Care System, Seattle, WA, and Department of Psychiatry and Behavioral Sciences, University of Washington, Seattle, WA.

Emily C. Williams is affiliated with Health Services Research & Development and Center of Excellence in Substance Abuse Treatment and Education, VA Puget Sound Health Care System, Seattle, WA and Departments of Medicine, and Health Services, University of Washington, Seattle, WA.

Steven M. Wright and Thomas Craig are affiliated with the Office of Quality and Performance, Veterans Health Administration, Washington, DC.

Katharine A. Bradley is affiliated with Health Services Research & Development, Primary and Specialty Medical Care, Center of Excellence in Substance Abuse Treatment and Education, VA Puget Sound Health Care System, Seattle, WA and the Departments of Medicine and Health Services, University of Washington, Seattle, WA.

Address correspondence to: Eric J. Hawkins, PhD, VA Puget Sound Health Care System-Seattle Division (S116ATC), 1660 South Columbian Way, Seattle, WA 98108 (E-mail: Eric.Hawkins@va.gov).

The research reported here was supported by Department of Veterans Affairs, Veterans Health Administration, Health Services Research and Development Service. The manuscript was specifically produced with support from the Veteran Affairs' Substance Use Disorders Quality Enhancement Research Initiative (SUB 98-000) and Center of Excellence in Substance Abuse Treatment & Education. Drs. Kivlahan and Bradley presently serve as the Clinical Coordinator and Co-Clinical Coordinator of the Substance Use Disorders Quality Enhancement Research Initiative.

The views expressed in this article are those of the authors and do not necessarily reflect the position or policy of the Department of Veterans Affairs or the University of Washington.

[Haworth co-indexing entry note]: "Examining Quality Issues in Alcohol Misuse Screening." Hawkins, Eric J. et al. Co-published simultaneously in *Substance Abuse* (The Haworth Medical Press, an imprint of The Haworth Press, Inc.) Vol. 28, No. 3, 2007, pp. 53-65; and: *Alcohol/ Drug Screening and Brief Intervention: Advances in Evidence-Based Practice* (ed: Richard Saitz, and Marc Galanter) The Haworth Medical Press, an imprint of The Haworth Press, Inc., 2007, pp. 53-65. Single or multiple copies of this article are available for a fee from The Haworth Document Delivery Service [1-800-HAWORTH, 9:00 a.m. - 5:00 p.m. (EST). E-mail address: docdelivery@haworthpress.com].

Available online at http://suba.haworthpress.com
doi:10.1300/J465v28n03_06

KEYWORDS. Alcohol screening, performance measure

INTRODUCTION

Alcohol misuse, including risky drinking and alcohol use disorders, is associated with considerable morbidity and mortality. Extensive research has documented the association between alcohol consumption and health problems (e.g., cancers, cardiovascular disorders, psychiatric disorders), and both unintentional and intentional deaths (1). Though the prevalence of alcohol use disorders in the US approximates 9%, the prevalence of risky alcohol use is greater with estimates as high as 30% in primary care settings (2, 3). Systematic reviews of brief intervention trials have concluded that brief interventions reduce risky drinking among outpatients (3). Recently, the National Commission on Prevention Priorities (NCPP) convened by the Partnership for Prevention and funded by the Agency for Healthcare Research and Quality and the Centers for Disease Control and Prevention identified alcohol screening and brief alcohol counseling among the top 10 national prevention priorities (4).

As a foundation for implementation of brief alcohol counseling (5), the Veterans Health Administration (VHA) implemented evidence-based alcohol misuse screening with the three Alcohol Use Disorders Identification Test Consumption Questions (AUDIT-C) in 2004. A recent report, comparing two independent methods for monitoring VHA performance for alcohol misuse screening, described the aggregate national results of the first year (2004) of alcohol misuse screening (6). Rates of screening and positive alcohol screens were estimated in two samples using two data sources: medical record reviews and patient surveys. The report described a high rate (93%) of alcohol misuse screening based on medical record reviews, suggesting successful implementation of evidence-based screening. However, there were differences between these complementary data sources in the prevalence of alcohol misuse.

The current study compared alcohol screening results documented in medical records and on patient surveys in a single sample of VHA outpatients to examine two general quality issues that arose during the first year routine alcohol misuse screening was implemented in the VHA. First, we compared AUDIT-C alcohol screening results documented clinically in the medical record and on mailed patient surveys. Second, we evaluated drinking practices reported on the AUDIT-C on mailed surveys among patients who were not screened clinically with the AUDIT-C because they had medical record documentation that they did not drink alcohol, they were participating in alcohol treatment, or they were screened with the full AUDIT.

METHODS

Background and Overview

Annual alcohol screening has been required in VHA since 1997, but prior to 2004 screening was performed primarily with the CAGE questionnaire, targeting patients with alcohol use disorders (6). In 2004, a national VHA performance measure was implemented that required screening for the broader spectrum of alcohol misuse (i.e., risky drinking or alcohol use disorders) with either the full 10-item Alcohol Use Disorders Identification Test (AUDIT) or the 3-item AUDIT-C.

In 2004, most alcohol misuse screening was conducted with the shorter AUDIT-C (6). Sites had considerable latitude on how they integrated alcohol screening into care (e.g., regarding who administered screening, how private the setting, etc.), but to facilitate implementation of the performance measure, a computerized clinical reminder for alcohol screening with the AUDIT-C was developed for the VHA's electronic medical record and disseminated nationally. To decrease the burden of unnecessary screening, patients who did not drink alcohol in the past year were not required to be screened. The clinical reminder prompted providers to indicate whether the patient drank alcohol in the past year, and if yes, to administer the AUDIT-C. The clinical reminder, which automatically calculated the AUDIT-C score, was widely implemented nationwide (6).

This is a cross-sectional study of VHA outpatients who participated in two quality improvement programs during this implementation period (2004). Patients were eligible if they both (1) had their clinical alcohol screening monitored by medical record review and (2) completed alcohol screening measures on mailed surveys. We analyzed concordance of screening results among this sample of patients who had screening data from both sources. Study approval was obtained from the University of Washington Human Subjects Committee and the VHA Office of Quality and Performance (OQP).

Data Collection

The VHA contracts with an external agency to conduct standardized medical record reviews of outpatient care as part of the External Peer Review Program (EPRP). In 2004 the VHA OQP randomly selected patients for review from each facility who had an outpatient visit in the previous month, over-sampling women so that they constituted approximately 25% of the sample (7). Patients receiving outpatient care associated with selected diagnostic conditions (e.g., coronary artery disease) were also over-sampled (7). Data from EPRP are used to monitor compliance with national VHA performance measures, which are used to determine salary incentives of directors and key managers of 21 regional VHA networks and 157 VHA medical centers.

Beginning in 2004, medical record reviews determined whether patients who were due for annual alcohol screening and drank alcohol in the past year were screened with the AUDIT-C or 10-item AUDIT. Alcohol screens performed prior to January 1, 2004 with previously approved screening measures (most sites used the CAGE which does not indicate whether patients currently drink alcohol) were acceptable until a patient was due for repeat annual alcohol screening. In lieu of screening, a provider could document that a patient did not drink alcohol, but in those situations medical record abstracters reviewed the medical record for the previous 12 months to confirm that there was not contradictory evidence in the medical record that the patient drank alcohol.

The Survey of Healthcare Experiences of Patients (SHEP) is mailed to selected VHA patients who had an outpatient visit in the previous month to support national quality improvement efforts and monitor patient satisfaction. During the first half of fiscal year 2004, SHEP included all outpatients sampled by EPRP and also randomly sampled established primary care patients. During the second half of 2004, a revised sampling strategy sampled patients equally from three groups: new primary care, established primary care, and specialty care. During this time, patients whose records were sampled by SHEP were sampled only coincidentally by EPRP. SHEP included items on alcohol use during eight months of 2004. The response rate for surveys mailed to outpatients during 2004 was approximately 70% (8).

Study Sample

Between October 1, 2003 and September 30, 2004, a total of 16,765 outpatients had their medical record reviewed by EPRP and returned a SHEP survey, which included a completed AUDIT-C. The VHA Alcohol Misuse Screening Performance Measure mandated that all outpatients receive annual alcohol screening with either the full 10-item AUDIT (9) or the 3-item AUDIT-C (10, 11). Several groups were not required to be screened clinically and, as a result, neither AUDIT nor AUDIT-C scores were available in the medical record for the following patient groups: those in palliative care or with documented cognitive impairment, those with provider documentation that they were nondrinkers of alcohol in the past year, and those with evidence of participation in alcohol treatment documented in the medical record in the past year.

Patients were potentially eligible for this study if they had their medical records reviewed for EPRP and completed the AUDIT-C on SHEP in fiscal year 2004 (N = 16,765). Potentially eligible patients were excluded from study analyses if they: (1) had no documentation of clinical screening for alcohol misuse (n = 968); (2) were screened clinically prior to January 1, 2004 with a previously acceptable screening measure other than AUDIT-C or AUDIT (most often the CAGE questionnaire) that did not indicate whether patients currently drank alcohol (n = 2,717); (3) had documented AUDIT-C screening but no AUDIT-C score recorded in the medical record (n = 570); (4) had documented 10-item AUDIT screening but no AUDIT score recorded in the medical record (n = 38); or (5) had a difference in clinical and survey alcohol screening dates that exceeded 365 days (N = 546). Figure 1 shows the number of patients excluded and screened with each instrument.

Measures

Data obtained from EPRP medical record reviews were used to ascertain: AUDIT-C score, full 10-item AUDIT score, non-drinking status, alcohol treatment participation, and screening date. In addition, data obtained from mailed SHEP surveys included AUDIT-C scores, return dates and demographic characteristics.

Clinically documented AUDIT-C. The AUDIT-C was used to screen for alcohol misuse by most VHA facilities in 2004. The AUDIT-C assesses alcohol consumption patterns in the past year and has been validated as a brief alcohol screening test in VHA (10, 12). Scores range from 0 to 12, with a cutoff of ≥ 4 and ≥ 3 identifying alcohol misuse in men and women, respectively. Higher AUDIT-C scores indicate greater alcohol misuse severity (11), and AUDIT-C scores of 8-12 have been associated with a higher risk for subsequent hospitalizations for liver disease, GI bleeding and pancreatitis (13), as well as mortality (14). Table 1 shows the AUDIT-C questions included in the widely disseminated alcohol screening clinical reminder used at many VHA facilities.

To facilitate interpretation of differences in clinically documented (EPRP) and survey (SHEP) AUDIT-C scores, we grouped respondents into four categories based on AUDIT-C scores: nondrinkers (AUDIT-C = 0), low-level drinkers who screen negative for alcohol misuse (AUDIT-C = 1-3 men; 1-2 women), mild-moderate alcohol misuse (AUDIT-C = 4-7 men; 3-7 women), and severe alcohol misuse (AUDIT-C = 8-12) (13).

Clinically documented nondrinkers. Patients with consistent documentation that they did not drink alcohol in the past year were exempt from required alcohol screening. If medical records indicated that patients did not drink alcohol, abstracters reviewed the medical record for the previous 12 months to confirm that

FIGURE 1. Development of study samples

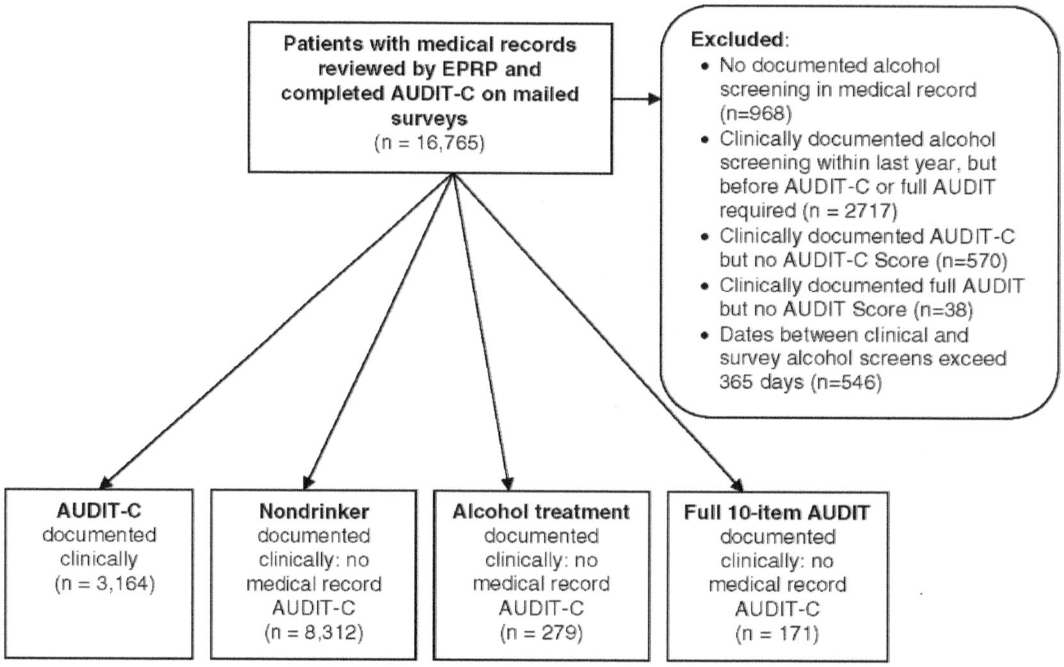

TABLE 1. The AUDIT-C Questions Included in the Widely Disseminated Clinical Reminder and SHEP Survey

AUDIT-C Screening Questionnaire in the Clinical Reminder

1. **How often did you have a drink containing alcohol in the past year?**
   Never (0 points), Monthly or less (1 point), Two to four times a month (2 points), Two to three times a week (3 points), Four or more times a week (4 points)

2. **How many drinks containing alcohol did you have on a typical day when you were drinking in the past year?**
   1 or 2 (0 points), 3 or 4 (1 point), 5 or 6 (2 points), 7 to 9 (3 points), 10 or more (4 points)

3. **How often did you have six or more drinks on one occasion in the past year?**
   Never (0 points), Less than monthly (1 point), Monthly (2 points), Weekly (3 points), Daily or almost daily (4 points)

Survey AUDIT-C Screening Questionnaire

1. **How often did you have a drink containing alcohol in the past 12 months? Consider a "drink" to be a can or bottle of beer, a glass of wine, a wine cooler, or one cocktail or a shot of hard liquor (like scotch, gin, or vodka).**
   Never (0 points), Monthly or less (1 point), 2-4 four times a month (2 points), 2-3 times a week (3 points), 4-5 times a week (4 points), 6 or more times a week (4 points)

2. **How many drinks containing alcohol did you have on a typical day when you were drinking in the past 12 months?**
   0 (0 points), 1-2 (0 points), 3-4 (1 point), 5-6 (2 points), 7-9 (3 points), 10 or more (4 points)

3. **How often did you have 6 or more drinks on one occasion in the past 12 months?**
   Never (0 points), Less than monthly (1 point), Monthly (2 points), Weekly (3 po ints), Daily or almost daily (4 points)

Scoring: Sum of scores for the 3 questions resulting in possible scores 0-12.

there was no evidence of alcohol consumption. In the event abstracters were unable to find a specific screening date to officially define the 12 month period under review, they were instructed to review the 12 months preceding the month in which the patient was sampled for EPRP review.

Clinically documented 10-item AUDIT. The 10-item AUDIT was developed by the WHO to identify patients with recent heavy drinking and alcohol abuse or dependence. The AUDIT is a reliable, well validated measure (9). AUDIT scores range from 0 to 40, with higher scores estimating greater alcohol misuse severity (15, 16). A screening cutoff score > 8 was used to identify alcohol misuse. Only a small number of patients were screened with the full AUDIT.

Clinically documented alcohol treatment. Patients were considered enrolled in alcohol treatment by EPRP, if medical record documentation indicated participation in a VHA or community-based treatment program or Alcoholics Anonymous. Patients with documentation of alcohol treatment at any time during the 12 month period preceding the date that their record was sampled by EPRP were not required to be screened for alcohol misuse.

Survey AUDIT-C. The AUDIT-C was included on SHEP for 8 months of 2004, and was used to calculate an AUDIT-C score (Table 1). To facilitate interpretation of differences in AUDIT-C scores documented in the medical record and those on the survey, we grouped AUDIT-C respondents into the same four categories outlined above.

Screening dates. The actual date that alcohol misuse screening was administered by a provider was abstracted from the medical record. The date of receipt by VHA was used as the screening date for surveys. Patients (n = 546) were excluded from the study, if the time between medical record and survey screening dates exceeded 365 days (see Figure 1). Although medical records were sampled for review during fiscal year 2004, the date of actual alcohol screening could have occurred any time in the preceding 12 months. Therefore, some screening was completed in 2003, leading to the possibility of differences in screening dates between clinical screening and survey screening that exceeded 365 days.

Definitions of discordance. Three types of discordance are discussed in this manuscript. They include discordance based on: (1) screening results, (2) drinking status, and (3) alcohol misuse severity. Discordance in screening results was defined as disagreement in alcohol misuse screening results between the data sources (e.g., clinically documented screen positive and survey screen negative). Discordance in drinking status was defined as disagreement between clinical documentation and survey report of alcohol use (e.g., drinker vs. nondrinker). An AUDIT-C score of 0 reflected no alcohol use in prior 12 months, whereas scores 1-12 indicate use of alcohol in the prior 12 months. Discordance in alcohol misuse severity was defined as clinical and survey AUDIT-C screening scores falling in different categories (defined above): nondrinker, low-level drinker, mild-moderate alcohol misuse, severe alcohol misuse.

Patient characteristics. The SHEP survey provided demographic data on self-reported race, marital status, education, employment status, and annual income. Patient age and gender were obtained from VHA administrative data files, and use of tobacco within the past 7 years was obtained from the medical record.

Analyses

Descriptive analyses were conducted to evaluate demographic characteristics of the four study samples based on clinical documentation: (1) patients screened with the AUDIT-C, (2) nondrinkers, (3) participants in alcohol treatment, and (4) patients screened with the full 10-item AUDIT. Statistical comparison of demographic characteristics of the groups were limited to nondrinkers and patients screened with the AUDIT-C, because of relatively small sample sizes of the patients in treatment and patients screened with the full 10-item AUDIT. We used chi-square and t-tests where appropriate for comparisons.

Our initial set of analyses examined differences in the screening prevalence and severity of alcohol misuse using the sample of patients screened with the AUDIT-C both clinically and by survey. Analyses were conducted in the following sequence. First, we compared screening results from the two data sources. Next, we used McNemar's chi-square test for paired data to test for a significant difference in screening results (positive vs. negative). Third, because we expected that discordance in screening results was associated with temporal differences in screening, we used logistic regression to test for an association between screening times and discordant screening status. To perform this analysis, differences between clinical and survey screening dates were categorized into three levels: 0 to 90 days, 91 to 180 days, and 181 to 365 days. Fourth, we repeated the analysis described in steps 1-2 using only cases that were screened within 90 days of each other (restricted sample). The remaining analyses were done with the restricted sample. Fifth, we conducted a multivariate logistic regression analysis to test for associations between demographic characteristics (age, gender, race, income, marital status) and tobacco use (use within past 7 years vs. no use) and discordant screening results between medical record and survey. Lastly, we used descriptive analysis and the intraclass correlation coefficient (ICC) to examine the degree of agreement between the medical record and survey AUDIT-C score categories and scores. The ICC analysis estimated the absolute agreement between medical record and survey AUDIT-C scores, using a single measurement, mixed model approach (17).

A second group of analyses used survey AUDIT-C scores to describe drinking patterns of three groups of patients not screened clinically with the AUDIT-C: patients documented to be nondrinkers, patients in alcohol treatment, and patients screened with the full AUDIT. First, we used descriptive analyses to evaluate the survey AUDIT-C in the clinically identified nondrinker sample, using the four AUDIT-C categories above. Next, we evaluated discordant drinking status (drinker vs. nondrinker) between the two sources using survey AUDIT-C results. For the nondrinker sample defined based on medical record review, the dates that patients' medical records were sampled for EPRP review were used to exclude patients whose medical record reviews were > 365 days apart from the date they returned SHEP, since only 29.6% of a total 8,716 nondrinkers had a specific date available when they were noted to be a nondrinker. Next, we used descriptive analyses to evaluate survey AUDIT-C responses among patients with clinical documentation of participation in alcohol treatment and screening with the 10-item AUDIT, using the four AUDIT-C categories above. In the latter sample of patients, we used McNemar's chi-square test to compare prevalence estimates of alcohol misuse using the clinically documented full AUDIT and survey AUDIT-C. Tests for the effect of time on screening results involving patients in treatment and patients screened with the 10 item AUDIT were not performed because sample sizes were insufficient to categorize time into multiple levels.

All analyses were performed using Intercooled Stata version 9.0 (18), with the exception of the calculation of ICC estimates, which were performed using SPSS version 13.0 (19).

RESULTS

Patient Characteristics

Demographic characteristics of the study samples are described in Table 2. Due to over-sampling of women in EPRP, women represent 20.5% of the clinically identified nondrinkers and 18.4% of the AUDIT-C screened sample in this study, considerably higher than the 6-7% of VHA patients in general who are women. Comparing the 3,164 patients with clinically documented screening with the AUDIT-C to the 8,312 patients clinically identified as nondrinkers, the latter were older by about one year on average: mean age 65.4 (SD = 12.4) vs. 66.6 (SD = 12.4), respectively ($p < 0.001$). Other demographic differences (i.e., gender, race, education, employment, and income) were statistically significant, but similarly small in magnitude. Medical record reviews preceded surveys for 91% of patients with clinically documented AUDIT-C screening (M = −108.3 days; SD = 105.9) and 95% of clinically documented nondrinkers (M = −113.9 days; SD = 102.5).

Prevalence of Alcohol Misuse Based on Medical Record Review and Surveys

Among patients with both clinically documented screening with the AUDIT-C and survey AUDIT-Cs, 20% reported no alcohol use in the past year and 45% reported low-level drinking on surveys (Table 3). The prevalence of alcohol misuse based on clinically documented AUDIT-Cs was 25.4% (CI: 23.9% to 26.9%) compared to 35.4% (CI: 32.7% to 36.0%) when the same patients were screened by AUDIT-C on survey (Table 4). The difference in prevalence rates was significant (diff = 9.0%; CI: 7.5% to 10.4%; $p < .001$). Screening results based on AUDIT-C screening documented in the medical record and surveys were discordant in 17.8% of patients, 75% (424/564) of whom screened positive on surveys and negative in clinically documented screening (Table 4).

We used logistic regression to test if the discordance in screening results (positive or negative) between clinical screening documented in the medical record and screening on mailed surveys was associated with the time between screening dates. Patients were categorized into three groups based on the number of days between medical record review and survey screening dates, 0-90 (n = 1637), 91-180 (n = 704), and 181-365 (n = 823) days. Patients with medical record review and survey screening dates within 0-90 days of each other represented the referent group. Patients whose medical record reviews and surveys were 91-180 days apart and 181-365 days apart, were more likely to have discordant alcohol screening results compared to patients with medical record review and survey screen dates within 90 days of each other [odds ratio (OR) = 1.41; CI: 1.13 to 1.77; $p < .01$, and OR = 1.32; CI: 1.06 to 1.64; $p < .05$, respectively]. As a result, further analyses were restricted to the 1,637 patients with clinically documented and survey AUDIT-C screening dates within 90 days of each other (M = 52.0 days, SD = 30.8). Among these patients, prevalence rates of positive screens in the medical record and on surveys were 24.6% (CI: 22.5% to 26.7%) and 33.4% (CI: 31.1% to 35.7%), respectively, and the difference in prevalence rates remained significant (diff = 8.8%; CI: 6.9% to 10.7%; $p < .001$). Using this restricted sample, a multivariate logistic re-

TABLE 2. Patient Characteristics of Four Samples Based on Clinical Documentation*

	AUDIT-C documented clinically (n = 3,164)		**Non-drinking documented clinically** (n = 8,312)		**Alcohol treatment documented clinically** (n = 279)		**10-item AUDIT documented clinically** (n = 171)	
Patient Characteristics	n	(%)	n	(%)	n	(%)	n	(%)
Age (year)††								
< 50	306	(9.7)	740	(8.9)	80	(28.7)	21	(12.3)
51-65	1187	(37.5)	2924	(35.2)	162	(58.1)	61	(35.7)
66-80	1319	(41.7)	3514	(42.3)	32	(11.5)	70	(40.9)
> 80	351	(11.1)	1134	(13.6)	5	(1.7)	19	(11.1)
Gender†								
Female	583	(18.4)	1688	(20.3)	39	(14.0)	43	(25.2)
Male	2581	(81.6)	6624	(79.7)	240	(86.0)	128	(74.8)
Ethnicity								
Non-Hispanic	2932	(96.1)	7741	(96.7)	248	(90.2)	148	(88.6)
Hispanic	118	(3.9)	251	(3.2)	24	(8.8)	19	(11.4)
Race††								
White	2740	(89.7)	7012	(87.2)	197	(72.4)	130	(80.8)
Black	205	(6.7)	685	(8.5)	44	(16.2)	29	(18.0)
Other	110	(3.6)	343	(4.3)	31	(11.4)	2	(1.2)
Marital Status††								
Divorced or separated	710	(23.0)	1682	(20.8)	136	(49.8)	33	(19.9)
Married	1882	(60.9)	4878	(60.2)	62	(22.7)	96	(57.8)
Widowed	300	(9.7)	932	(11.5)	24	(8.8)	23	(13.9)
Never married	198	(6.4)	610	(7.5)	51	(18.7)	14	(8.4)
Education†††								
High school or less	1402	(45.3)	4375	(54.0)	121	(43.9)	70	(42.4)
Some college	985	(31.8)	2369	(29.3)	116	(42.0)	51	(30.9)
College or beyond	709	(22.9)	1354	(16.7)	39	(14.1)	44	(26.7)
Employment†††								
Retired	1692	(54.5)	4518	(55.6)	63	(23.1)	81	(48.8)
Unable to work	596	(19.2)	2091	(25.7)	126	(46.1)	42	(25.3)
Employed	657	(21.2)	1157	(14.2)	48	(17.6)	35	(21.1)
Unemployed	86	(2.8)	166	(2.0)	28	(10.3)	5	(3.0)
Other	72	(2.3)	200	(2.5)	8	(2.9)	3	(1.8)
Income (k)†††								
< 30	2094	(70.8)	6172	(80.0)	235	(88.0)	114	(73.1)
30 – 60	662	(22.4)	1300	(16.9)	29	(10.9)	36	(23.1)
> 60	201	(6.8)	243	(3.1)	3	(1.0)	6	(3.8)

* Samples are defined based on EPRP Medical Record Reviews and data are from SHEP surveys (except age and gender); data exclude missing values for patient characteristics, because not all respondents answered every question on surveys.

† $p < 0.05$

†† $p < 0.01$

††† $p < 0.001$

TABLE 3. Survey Alcohol Misuse Screening Results

	AUDIT-C documented clinically (n = 3164)		Non-drinking documented clinically (n = 8,312)		Alcohol treatment documented clinically (n = 279)		10-item AUDIT documented clinically (n = 171)	
	n	(%)	n	(%)	n	(%)	n	(%)
Survey AUDIT-C (score)								
Nondrinker (0)	651	(20.6)	6343	(76.3)	121	(43.4)	49	(28.7)
Screen negative (1-3)	1125	(45.0)	1582	(19.0)	32	(11.5)	59	(34.5)
Mild/Moderate Alcohol Misuse (4-7)[a]	901	(28.5)	339	(4.1)	66	(23.6)	50	(29.2)
Severe alcohol misuse (8-12)	187	(5.9)	48	(0.6)	60	(21.5)	13	(7.6)

[a] Because AUDIT-C cutoff for women is ≥ 3, women with a score = 3 are included in this category.

TABLE 4. Alcohol Misuse Screening Rate Comparison Between Medical Record and Survey Based on Sample Screened with AUDIT-C (n = 3,164)

	Self-Report Survey					
	+ Screen	**(%)**	**- Screen**	**(%)**	**Total**	**(%)**
Medical Record						
+ Screen	664	(21.0)	140	(4.4)	804	(25.4)
- Screen	424	(13.4)	1936	(61.2)	2360	(74.6)
	1088	(34.4)	2076	(65.6)	3164	(100.0)

gression model was used to determine demographic and clinical factors associated with discordant screening results between the two data sources. Variables included in the model were age, gender, race, income, marital status and tobacco use. The odds of discordant screening results were increased only among users of tobacco within the past 7 years (OR = 1.41; CI: 1.05 to 1.89; $p < .05$).

The ICC estimate measuring the degree of agreement between clinically documented and survey AUDIT-C scores for patients screened within 90 days was 0.67 (CI: .61 to .72), representing a "good" level of agreement (20). Figure 2 depicts AUDIT-C scores documented in the medical record (bars) in groups defined based on AUDIT-C scores on surveys (horizontal axis). The consistency between medical record and survey AUDIT-C scores was highest for low-level drinkers who screened negative for alcohol misuse (AUDIT-C 1-3), with over 80% of patients whose surveys indicated this level of drinking having consistent results documented clinically. In contrast, less than a third of patients scoring within the 8-12 range on the survey AUDIT-C were found to have scores within this range based on clinically documented screening with the AUDIT-C.

Patients Who Were Not Screened Clinically with the AUDIT-C

Table 3 shows survey AUDIT-C responses for patients who were not screened clinically with the AUDIT-C because medical record documentation indicated they were non-drinkers (n = 8,312), were in alcohol treatment (n = 279) or were screened instead with the full 10-item AUDIT (n = 171). Survey AUDIT-C scores of patients identified as nondrinkers in the medical record review showed that 24% were discordant and self-reported alcohol consumption in the past year, with 5% (CI: 4.2% to 5.1%) screening positive for alcohol misuse on surveys. The mean difference in days between screening dates for medical record and survey was 113.3 days (SD = 102.5). Among patients clinically documented as receiving alcohol treatment, 57% reported drinking in the past year, and 45% (CI: 39.3% to 51.0%) screened positive for alcohol misuse on the AUDIT-C on surveys. Among 171 patients with medical record documentation of screening with the 10-item AUDIT, only 9 (5%) screened positive at the specified threshold (≥ 8), although of those who screened negative (n = 162), 33% screened positive on the survey AUDIT-C: 45

FIGURE 2. Comparison of medical record and survey AUDIT-C score categories restricted to patients screened within 90 days (n = 1,637)

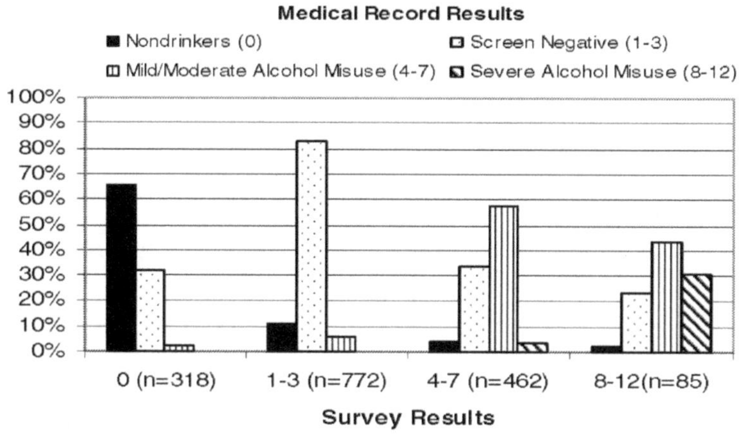

(27.7%) with AUDIT-C scores of 4-7 and 9 (5.6%) with AUDIT-C scores of 8-12. The prevalence of alcohol misuse based on the medical record 10-item AUDIT (5.3%; CI: 1.9% to 8.6%) and survey AUDIT-C (36.8%; CI: 29.5%t o 44.1%) differed significantly (diff = 31.6%; CI: 24.0% to 39.1%; $p < 0.001$) using standard cutoffs (AUDIT $\geq$ 8; AUDIT-C $\geq$ 4 for men and $\geq$ 3 for women).

DISCUSSION

This study compared clinical alcohol screening results to screening with the same instrument included on mailed surveys and found that the prevalence of alcohol misuse was significantly lower when assessed clinically. Moreover, this difference remained when analyses were restricted to patients screened clinically and by survey within three months of each other. About 18% of patients had discordant alcohol screening results based on clinical and survey screening, and 75% of these patients with discordant results screened negative in clinical screening and positive on surveys. In addition, 24% of patients identified as nondrinkers in the medical record (and therefore not screened clinically), self-reported drinking in the past year on mailed surveys, and 5% screened positive for alcohol misuse.

The goal of alcohol misuse screening is to identify patients with alcohol misuse so that providers can offer patients brief alcohol counseling and make appropriate referrals to treatment. A previously published report noted that the VHA successfully implemented evidenced-based alcohol misuse screening in 2004, but also that rates of alcohol misuse based on medical record review and surveys suggested potentially important variation (6). However, that study compared clinical alcohol screening documented in the medical record and mailed surveys in different samples. The discrepancy between medical record and survey prevalence rates of alcohol misuse in that study also called into question the appropriateness of excluding certain groups of patients from clinical alcohol screening. This study extends the prior report by comparing survey and medical record alcohol screening results in the same sample.

Self-report surveys typically identify more alcohol misuse and are likely more accurate than clinical interviews for several reasons (21, 22). Surveys used for research or quality improvement purposes, like the one used in this study, typically provide patients with assurances of confidentiality that clinical interviews do not, which may have resulted in the differences in alcohol use and misuse found in this study. Alcohol screening questionnaires administered by interview are more likely to be biased by social desirability (23). While interviewers can help motivate patients to honestly answer questions, several factors are essential for promoting accurate reporting on alcohol screening: asking questions verbatim, in a private setting, and in a nonjudgmental manner

(24). In primary care settings providers may be uncomfortable with alcohol-related discussions (25, 26), potentially leading to discomfort on the part of patients. In addition, patients may underestimate alcohol use because of perceived stigma associated with alcohol misuse. Of note, the heaviest drinkers, patients with AUDIT-C scores 8-12 based on surveys had the greatest discordance in AUDIT-C categories, with only 30% also having AUDIT-C scores in that range based on clinical screening documented in the medical record.

It is important to note that the alcohol misuse prevalence rates reported in this study do not accurately describe the population-based prevalence of alcohol misuse found in the VHA. The random sample used in this study over-sampled women and patients with diagnostic conditions who are less likely to use or misuse alcohol. However, the difference between prevalence rates found in this study is important, and our findings suggest a need for further refinement of the VHA's screening procedures for alcohol misuse. In response, the VHA has enacted a number of changes to its alcohol screening. Results of a recent validation study comparing the AUDIT-C to an interview "gold" standard of alcohol misuse found no change in the cutoff score (≥ 4) when using an imputed AUDIT-C score of 0 for patients who reported never drinking on question #1 (27). Thus, one of the changes to VHA alcohol misuse screening includes requiring that all patients, except those who are terminally ill or cognitively impaired, be screened for alcohol misuse with the validated first question of the AUDIT-C. If patients respond to AUDIT-C question #1, which assesses how often they drank alcohol in the past year, by indicating "never," an AUDIT-C score of 0 can be imputed without asking the other two questions (27). An electronic clinical reminder has been updated to incorporate this requirement. The VHA has addressed under-detection of alcohol misuse by promoting a number of specific strategies designed to further standardize interview screening procedures. These include requiring documentation of patient responses to each AUDIT-C item to encourage providers to ask questions verbatim and encouraging providers to conduct screening in confidential settings (e.g., exam room) and in a nonjudgmental manner to minimize the effects of social desirability bias (28).

In 2004, patients in VHA or community-based alcohol treatment were excluded from the VHA's annual alcohol screening requirement because screening was not considered necessary in patients with known alcohol use disorders. Unsurprisingly, in a small sample of patients not screened clinically because of alcohol treatment participation, survey responses showed 45% screened positive for alcohol misuse in the past year. However, the implications of this finding are unclear because medical record abstraction did not indicate when or for how long these patients participated in VHA or community based treatment, or whether the AUDIT-C results represent a period of time before or since treatment was initiated. Regardless, annual alcohol screening for patients in alcohol treatment would create an opportunity for providers to assess and support patient treatment engagement and response. For these reasons, the VHA now requires annual alcohol screening regardless of treatment status.

This study also suggested 33% of patients who screen negative with the 10-item AUDIT at a screening threshold of ≥ 8, screen positive for alcohol misuse using the AUDIT-C at the standard threshold (≥ 4 men/≥ 3 women), and 6% had AUDIT-C scores of 8-12 reflecting severe misuse. This is consistent with validation studies in VHA and non-VHA outpatients in the US, suggesting that the standard screening threshold of ≥ 8 for the full AUDIT has low sensitivity for alcohol misuse in US outpatient populations (27, 29). Moreover, this finding–that using different validated alcohol misuse screening tests can identify very different samples–indicates the importance of standardizing alcohol screening questionnaires and thresholds for assessing the targeted population for brief alcohol counseling (6). As a result, the VHA now requires the use of the AUDIT-C to screen for alcohol misuse.

This study has several limitations. Both the medical record and survey AUDIT-C scores are based on patient self-report. Though self-report is considered a reliable and valid approach to measurement of alcohol consumption (24, 30, 31), it is also subject to a number of biases (31). These biases may have underestimated or overestimated true patterns of alcohol use.

Moreover, this study did not include a "gold standard" interview measure for assessing alcohol consumption. It is also possible that differences in the clinical and survey AUDIT-C measures (see Table 1) contributed to the differences in screening results found in this study. The survey defined standard drink sizes and asked specifically about the past 12 months instead of the less precise "past year." In addition, the commonly used clinical reminder did not use a validated question to assess alcohol use. Further, the generalizability of our findings may be limited, because the study sample is comprised primarily of older, white men of lower socioeconomic status. The sampling strategy used to sample outpatients' medical records was not completely random. Oversampling of women and selected diagnostic conditions may have included patients less likely to use or misuse alcohol. In addition, the sampling strategy used for the surveys was revised during 2004 and survey data were available for only eight of the 12 months, which may have further limited the generalizability of our findings. It is possible that provider and facility characteristics contribute to discordance rates found in this study, but this study was not able to examine these associations. Additionally, although our analyses assessed the effect of time between clinical and survey screening on discordant outcomes, and restricted analyses to those within three months of each other, assessments were not concurrent. Therefore, time may still confound our analyses and some discordant outcomes may accurately reflect changes in drinking. Finally, this study cannot address specific reasons patients report lower levels of drinking when screened clinically compared to when screened by self-administered surveys. Despite these limitations, this is the first study to our knowledge to compare alcohol screening conducted as part of routine clinical practice to alcohol screening on patient surveys. These analyses of alcohol screening in the largest integrated health care system in the US have important implications for health care systems considering implementing similar alcohol screening programs, as a prelude to implementation of brief alcohol counseling.

These findings emphasize the importance of measuring the quality of clinical alcohol misuse screening as well as the proportion of patients who are screened for alcohol misuse. Despite the successful implementation of alcohol misuse screening, this study suggests that some alcohol misuse remains undetected by clinical alcohol screening. Whereas assessment of the prevalence of alcohol misuse screening can suggest variation in quality and under-detection of alcohol misuse by clinical screening (6), direct comparison of clinical screening results to mailed surveys is a more direct measure of quality. Efforts like those currently underway in the VHA are likely necessary to improve the quality of screening when it occurs. Additionally, the results of this study support systematic screening of nondrinkers and patients who are referred to alcohol treatment, and show the importance of using a single alcohol screening questionnaire to assess alcohol misuse.

In conclusion, we compared clinically documented alcohol screening to responses to the same screening questionnaire on mailed surveys and found that the prevalence of alcohol misuse among VHA patients is likely underestimated in clinical alcohol screening. These findings emphasize the importance of the quality and standardization of alcohol misuse screening. The VHA has therefore modified its performance measure for alcohol screening to further improve the quality and standardization of screening as the foundation for efforts to improve brief alcohol counseling.

REFERENCES

1. Room R, Babor T, Rehm J. Alcohol and public health. Lancet. 2005;365(9458):519-30.
2. Saitz R. Clinical practice. Unhealthy alcohol use. N Engl J Med. 2005;352(6):596-607.
3. Whitlock EP, Polen MR, Green CA, Orleans T, Klein J. Behavioral counseling interventions in primary care to reduce risky/harmful alcohol use by adults: A summary of the evidence for the U.S. Preventive Services Task Force. Ann Intern Med. 2004;140:557-568.
4. Maciosek MV, Coffield AB, Edwards NM, Flottemesch TJ, Goodman MJ, Solberg LI. Priorities among effective clinical preventive services results of a systematic review and analysis. Am J Prev Med. 2006; 31(1):52-61.
5. Babor TE, Higgins-Biddle J, Dauser D, Higgins P, Burleson JA. Alcohol screening and brief intervention in primary care settings: implementation models and predictors. J Stud Alcohol. 2005;66(3):361-8.

6. Bradley KA, Williams EC, Achtmeyer CE, Volpp B, Collins BJ, Kivlahan DR. Implementation of evidence-based alcohol screening in the Veterans Health Administration. Am J Manag Care. 2006;12(10):597-606.

7. EPRP Technical Manual. http://vaww.oqp.med.va.gov/ 2004.

8. Wright SM, Craig T, Campbell S, Schaefer J, Humble C. Patient satisfaction of female and male users of Veterans Health Administration services. J Gen Intern Med. 2006;21 Suppl 3:S26-32.

9. Saunders JB, Aasland OG, Babor TF, De la Fuente JR, Grant M. Development of the Alcohol Use Disorders Identification Test (AUDIT): WHO collaborative project on early detection of persons with harmful alcohol consumption–II. Addiction. 1993;88:791-804.

10. Bush KR, Kivlahan DR, McDonell MB, Fihn SD, Bradley KB. The AUDIT alcohol consumption questions (AUDIT-C): an effective brief screening test for problem drinking. Arch Intern Med. 1998;158: 1789-1795.

11. Bradley KA, Kivlahan DR, Zhou XH, et al. Using alcohol screening results and treatment history to assess the severity of at-risk drinking in VA primary care patients. Alcohol Clin Exp Res. 2004;28(3):448-455.

12. Bradley KA, Bush K, Davis TD, et al. Two brief alcohol screening tests from the Alcohol Use Disorders Identification Test (AUDIT): validation in a female VA patient population. Arch Intern Med. 2003;163:821-839.

13. Au DH, Kivlahan DR, Bryson CL, Blough D, Bradley KA. Alcohol screening scores and risk of hospitalizations for GI conditions in men. Alcohol Clin Exp Res. 2007;31(3):1-9.

14. Bradley KA, Maynard C, Kivlahan DR, McDonell MB, Fihn SD. The relationship between alcohol screening questionnaires and mortality among male veteran outpatients. J Stud Alcohol. 2001;62(6):826-33.

15. Babor TF, Higgins-Biddle JC, Saunders JB, Monteiro MG. AUDIT: The Alcohol Use Disorders Identification Test: Guidelines for Use in Primary Care, 2nd Edition, http://www.dass.stir.ac.uk/DRUGS/pdf/audit.pdf. In: World Health Organization DoMHaSD, ed; 2001.

16. Donovan DM, Kivlahan DR, Doyle SR, Longabaugh R, Greenfield SF. Concurrent validity of the Alcohol Use Disorders Identification Test (AUDIT) and AUDIT zones in defining levels of severity among out-patients with alcohol dependence in the COMBINE study. Addiction. 2006;101(12):1696-704.

17. McGraw KO, Wong SP. Forming inferences about some intraclass correlation coefficients. Psychological Methods. 1996;1:30-46.

18. Intercooled Stata 9.2 for Windows. College Station, TX: StataCorp; 2006.

19. Statistical Package for the Social Sciences for Windows Version 13.0.1 (computer program). Chicago: SPSS, Inc.; 2004.

20. Cicchetti DV. Guidelines, criteria, and rules of thumb for evaluating normed and standardized assessment instruments in psychology. Psychological Assessment. 1994;6:284-290.

21. Gmel G. The effect of mode of data collection and of non-response on reported alcohol consumption: a split-sample study in Switzerland. Addiction. 2000;95(1): 123-34.

22. Kraus L, Augustin R. Measuring alcohol consumption and alcohol-related problems: comparison of responses from self-administered questionnaires and telephone interviews. Addiction. 2001;96(3):459-71.

23. Bowling A. Mode of questionnaire administration can have serious effects on data quality. J Public Health (Oxf). 2005;27(3):281-91.

24. Del Boca FK, Noll JA. Truth or consequences: the validity of self-report data in health services research on addictions. Addiction. 2000;95 Suppl 3:S347-60.

25. Aira M, Kauhanen J, Laricaara P, Rautio P. Factors influencing inquiry about patients' alcohol consumption by primary health care physicians: qualitative semi-structured interview study. Fam Practice. 2003; 20(3):270-275.

26. McCormick KA, Cochran NE, Back AL, Merrill JO, Williams EC, Bradley KA. How Primary Care Providers Talk to Patients about Alcohol: A Qualitative Study. J Gen Intern Med. 2006;21:966-972.

27. Bradley KA, DeBenedetti AF, Volk RJ, Williams EC, Frank D, Kivlahan DR. AUDIT-C as a brief screen for alcohol misuse in primary care. Alcohol Clin Exp Res. 2007;31:1208-1217.

28. EPRP Technical Manual. http://vaww.oqp.med.va.gov/ 2007;accessed November, 2006.

29. Volk RJ, Steinbauer JR, Cantor SB, Holzer CEI. The Alcohol Use Disorders Identification Test (AUDIT) as a screen for at-risk patients of different racial/ethnic backgrounds. Addiction. 1997;92(2):197-206.

30. Babor TF, DelBoca FK. Just the Facts: enhancing measurement of alcohol consumption using self report methods. In: Litten RZ, Allen JP, eds. Measuring alcohol consumption. Totowa: Humana Press; 1992: 3-19.

31. Del Boca FK, Darkes J. The validity of self-reports of alcohol consumption: state of the science and challenges for research. Addiction. 2003;98 Suppl 2:1-12.

doi:10.1300/J465v28n03_06

The Cost-Effectiveness and Cost-Benefit of Screening and Brief Intervention for Unhealthy Alcohol Use in Medical Settings

Kevin L. Kraemer, MD, MSc

SUMMARY. Economic evaluation can be a valuable tool for assessing the efficiency and value of health care programs. To examine the literature on the economic evaluation of alcohol screening and brief intervention in medical settings, relevant studies were identified in the MEDLINE database (1966 through November 2006) and by hand-searching the references of identified articles and relevant journals. The 15 identified studies used a range of economic evaluation methods, including cost analysis, cost-benefit, cost-effectiveness, and cost-utility. Nearly all of the studies supported the use of alcohol screening and brief intervention. The studies that prospectively collected cost and effect data and/or conformed closely to methodological guidelines demonstrated a strong economic benefit of alcohol screening and brief intervention when compared to usual care. Overall, the reviewed studies support alcohol SBI in medical settings as a wise use of health care resources and illustrate the usefulness of economic evaluation for assessing alcohol prevention and treatment programs. doi:10.1300/J465v28n03_07

KEYWORDS. Alcohol, screening, economic evaluation, cost-benefit, cost-effectiveness

INTRODUCTION

The great societal burden from alcohol is potentially lessened by screening and brief intervention (SBI) for unhealthy alcohol use in medical settings (1-5). However, because alcohol SBI must compete with numerous other health conditions for provider time and limited health care resources, even efficacious approaches to alcohol SBI may not be implemented nor adequately funded by insurers (6). Future constraints on resources could further jeopardize the delivery of many health care services, including those targeted at unhealthy alcohol use.

Kevin L. Kraemer is affiliated with the Center for Research on Health Care, Division of General Internal Medicine, University of Pittsburgh School of Medicine, Pittsburgh, PA.

Address correspondence to: Kevin L. Kraemer, MD, MSc, Center for Research on Health Care, Division of General Internal Medicine, University of Pittsburgh School of Medicine, 230 McKee Place, Suite 600, Pittsburgh, PA 15213 (E-mail: kraemerkl@upmc.edu).

Support for this work was provided by the National Institute on Alcohol Abuse and Alcoholism (grant AA14713) and the National Institute on Drug Abuse (grant DA18139).

[Haworth co-indexing entry note]: "The Cost-Effectiveness and Cost-Benefit of Screening and Brief Intervention for Unhealthy Alcohol Use in Medical Settings." Kraemer, Kevin L. Co-published simultaneously in *Substance Abuse* (The Haworth Medical Press, an imprint of The Haworth Press, Inc.) Vol. 28, No. 3, 2007, pp. 67-77; and: *Alcohol/Drug Screening and Brief Intervention: Advances in Evidence-Based Practice* (ed: Richard Saitz, and Marc Galanter) The Haworth Medical Press, an imprint of The Haworth Press, Inc., 2007, pp. 67-77. Single or multiple copies of this article are available for a fee from The Haworth Document Delivery Service [1-800-HAWORTH, 9:00 a.m. - 5:00 p.m. (EST). E-mail address: docdelivery@haworthpress.com].

Available online at http://suba.haworthpress.com

doi:10.1300/J465v28n03_07

Therefore, alcohol programs such as SBI in medical settings must not only be effective but also "cost-effective."

Economic evaluation is a valuable tool for assessing the efficiency and value of health care programs and is an important input to resource allocation decisions (7-10). There are several excellent methodological reviews of economic evaluation for alcohol treatment programs (11-13). While extensive work has been done on the costs and benefits of treatment for alcohol dependence (14-24), economic analyses focused on SBI in medical settings for non-dependent unhealthy alcohol use are much less common. This report will briefly review common types of economic evaluation used in health care and summarize published economic studies of SBI for unhealthy alcohol use in different medical settings.

Types of Economic Evaluation

Several economic evaluation methods can be used to compare the costs and outcomes of health care programs. Straightforward *cost analysis* of a program's direct health care costs compared to an alternative program (8) is common but is considered only a partial economic evaluation because it does not take the health outcomes of a program into account. In contrast, full economic evaluation simultaneously compares the costs and health outcomes of two or more alternative programs. Full economic evaluation in health care typically uses the following analytic approaches: (1) cost-minimization analysis; (2) cost-benefit analysis; (3) cost-effectiveness analysis; and (4) cost-utility analysis (8). *Cost-Minimization Analysis* (CMA) is used for comparing programs that produce equivalent health outcomes. In such cases, the analysis simply seeks to determine the least costly of the alternative programs which are assumed equally efficacious. The program that is least costly is favored because it offers a better value (e.g., more "health" per dollar spent).

Cost-Benefit Analysis (CBA) measures both the opportunity costs and benefits (outcomes) of a health care program in monetary terms. (10,25) The result of a CBA study is often presented as a dimensionless benefit-cost ratio (e.g., health benefits divided by costs) where a value greater than 1 indicates the benefits of a program exceed the costs. Although uncommonly used in the past for analysis of health care programs because it requires the sometimes difficult conversion of outcomes into monetary terms, CBA has several strengths that render it an attractive methodology (8,26). First, CBA is ideally a comprehensive analysis of all costs and benefits of a program. Second, CBA has a strong theoretical foundation in welfare economics (25). Third, CBA is well-suited for decision-making because the value of a program (e.g., is it *worth* the costs?) is apparent if the analysis is well-done. CBA has appeal for the analysis of alcohol and drug treatment programs because some of the diverse outcomes of treatment, such as crime, employment, and societal well-being, are external to the health benefit to the individual alcohol or drug user and are difficult to incorporate into other types of economic evaluation (11,26,28,29). However, CBA is limited by the challenge of valuing health and non-health outcomes, such as quality-of-life benefits to substance users, their family members and friends, and to others in society.

A type of partial CBA, the *cost-offset study*, is perhaps the most commonly used and reported type of economic analysis of alcohol treatment (14-17). Cost offsets are net reductions in direct health care costs attributable to alcoholism treatment. While providing useful information, the cost-offset approach is not particularly useful for decision-making because it considers a relatively narrow set of outcomes (avoided direct health care costs) (26). Methods for the CBA of alcohol programs have been improving (11-13,26).

Cost-Effectiveness Analysis (CEA) is used to compare the relative value of alternative programs for creating better health and/or longer life. The results of such evaluations are usually summarized as cost-effectiveness (CE) ratios, where costs in the numerator are related to some single, common measure of effectiveness in the denominator (7-10). The effectiveness term may be life years gained or some pertinent clinical marker (e.g., abstinence from alcohol at one year). The incremental CE ratio indicates the marginal health effect gained by spending dollars on a program compared to an alternative program, and is expressed as cost per unit of effect (e.g., dollars per life year saved; dollars per abstinent year).

Cost-Utility Analysis (CUA) is a special form of CEA where health-related quality of life is integrated into the effectiveness term (7). CUA follows from the recognition that "health" is not simply about maximizing survival but is also related to functioning in key domains such as physical, psychological, and social/role function, health perceptions, and symptoms (31,32). Quality-Adjusted Life Years (QALYs) are the recommended effectiveness measure (denominator) for CUA (7,33). QALYs are a composite measure reflecting the product of quantity of life (e.g., survival, life expectancy) and health-related quality of life. The health-related quality of life term is typically a preference-based utility measure that is interval scaled from zero (poorest health state or death) to one (full health), such that a year of life in full health is equal to 1 QALY whereas a year of life with a health utility of 0.8 is equal to 0.8 QALYs (7,8). QALYs are calculated by multiplying the time an individual (real or hypothetical) spends in a specific health state by the utility weight for that health state, summing over all the health states that the individual experiences over the time horizon of interest, and then aggregating over the population under examination. The incremental CE ratio for CUA is expressed as cost per QALY gained. CUA is the preferred method for evaluation when health-related quality of life is a key outcome for the disease state in question (7).

CUA is the recommended method of the U.S. Public Health Service Panel on Cost-Effectiveness in Health and Medicine (7). However, there are few published economic evaluations of alcohol programs that use QALYs as the effectiveness measure. This is a potential limitation to the field because CUA is perhaps the fasting growing and most used of the types of economic evaluation (7,34). CUA is a standard, well-accepted technique for comparing health care programs and has had significant influence on policy for spectrum of health conditions, including coronary artery disease (35-37), stroke (38), and HIV disease (39), and is becoming the standard for evaluating new pharmaceutical products (40-42).

However, CUA does have limitations related to evaluation of alcohol programs. First, both CEA and CUA provide the incremental cost to achieve some goal (e.g., life-year gained, QALY gained) but do not indicate whether achieving the goal is *worth* the costs. To do so, CEA and CUA must use some external criterion value for the analyses to be useful for decision-making and resource allocation. Because the oft-quoted external criterion threshold of $50,000-$100,000 per QALY range is not based on empirical data, determination of society's willingness-to-pay to gain a QALY is an area that requires investigation or at least frequent reassessment (43,44). Second, some analysts have questioned the appropriateness of CUA for the evaluation of alcohol programs because the diverse outcomes of alcohol use external to the individual cannot be captured in the single metric of QALYs (11,26,45). However, CUA can account for changes in crime, health care utilization, and employment as cost savings in the numerator of the cost-effectiveness (CE) ratio (7,8,46). Furthermore, even in the absence of accounting for external non-health benefits of alcohol treatment, CUA has the advantage of producing a common metric (e.g., dollars per QALY) that is now available for numerous interventions, pharmaceuticals, and screening procedures for a broad spectrum of health conditions (34).

Economic Evaluations of SBI for Unhealthy Alcohol Use

To examine the literature on the economic evaluation of alcohol SBI in medical settings, all relevant studies were identified by searching the MEDLINE database (1966 through November 2006) for the terms cost-effectiveness, cost-benefit, economic evaluation, alcohol, screening, and brief intervention and by hand-searching the references of identified articles and relevant journals.

Table 1 summarizes 15 published economic evaluations of SBI for unhealthy alcohol use in 3 medical settings: primary care, inpatient, and the emergency department (ED). Except for cost-minimization analysis, each of the economic evaluation techniques described in the previous section is represented in Table 1. Some studies (47-49) are partial cost analyses, each describing the costs of implementing and conducting an alcohol screening and/or BI pro-

TABLE 1. Summary of Published Economic Evaluations for Alcohol SBI. The Focus of the Studies Is on Unhealthy Alcohol Use. The Results for Many of These Studies Were Initially Reported in Non-US Currency. With the Exception of Chisholm et al. (54), All Costs Have Been Converted to US Dollars for the Appropriate Year.

Clinical Setting	Study	Year	Type of Analysis	Strategy Comparisons	Findings	Comments
Primary Care						
	King (62)	1986	CBA: threshold analysis within cross-sectional study	Screening with CAGE vs. no screening	Screening with CAGE is worthwhile if the benefit of detecting 1 at-risk drinker is at least 1.89 times the cost of a false positive	• Target population: primary care patients • Not a true CBA because monetary valuation of costs and benefits not required for this analysis
	Lindholm (50)	1998	CEA: computer simulation	1) PCP-delivered BI (5 visits over 1 year) vs. no BI 2) Nurse-delivered BI (5 visits over 1 year) vs. no BI	PCP and Nurse alcohol advice is cost saving even if only 10% sustained a change from heavy to moderate drinking	• Target population: "heavy drinkers" in primary care screened with CAGE • Alcohol advice was cost-effective even when efficacy was very low (1-2% sustained change from heavy to moderate drinking)
	Fleming et al. (51)	2000	CBA: analysis within RCT	PCP-delivered BI (2 15-minute sessions plus 2 phone follow-ups) vs. no BI	Savings of $5.63 for every $1.00 spent on BI	• Target population: primary care problem drinkers (> 14 drinks/week in men and > 11 drinks/week in women) • Each arm of study was screened • Based on 12-month follow-up data from Project TrEAT,(3) a 48-month study
	Wutzke et al. (52)	2001	CEA: computer simulation	1) PCP-delivered BI (5 minutes) with minimal training support vs. no BI 2) PCP-delivered BI with maximal training support vs. PCP-delivered BI with minimal training support	$974 per life year saved for BI $1492 per life year saved for BI with maximal support	• Target population: "at-risk" drinkers in primary care • Costs included tele-marketing the SBI package to PCPs (Gomel, et al. 1998) (63) • Minimal training support was defined as 5 minutes initial training plus advice to clinic receptionist biweekly • Maximal training support was 5 minutes initial training plus alternate telephone and clinic visits biweekly
	Fleming et al. (53)	2002	CBA: analysis within RCT	PCP-delivered BI (2 15-minute sessions plus 2 phone follow-ups) vs. no BI	Savings of $4.30 for every $1.00 spent on BI	• 48-month follow-up data from Project TrEAT (3) described above
	Kaner et al. (47)	2003	Cost analysis: analysis within RCT	3 strategies to encourage primary care nurses to perform SBI for alcohol: 1) Outreach training 2) Training plus telephone support 3) Written guidelines	1) $47.79 per BI delivered 2) $46.50 per BI delivered	• Costs collected prospectively at 212 practices • Did not report incremental cost-effectiveness ratios

				(control group)	3) $47.79 per BI delivered	
	Chisholm et al. (54)	2004	CUA: state-transition population model	PCP–delivered BI (4 primary care visits over 1 year) vs. no BI (assumed current taxation on alcohol)	In US and Canada, BI costs I$24,073 per DALY averted	• Target population: hazardous drinkers (> 40 grams ethanol/day for men, >20 grams ethanol/day for women) • Assumed 50% of hazardous drinkers were targeted for BI and adherence of 70% in those targeted (i.e., 35% of hazardous drinking population received BI) • I$ = international dollars, a hypothetical unit of currency that reflects the worth of a country's currency within the country's borders
	Andrews et al. (55)	2004	CEA: computer simulation	1) Evidence-based BI with current coverage (8%) vs. no BI 2) Evidence-based BI with optimal coverage (70%) vs. no BI	1) $6,593 per YLD averted for BI with current coverage 2) $10,250 per YLD averted for BI with optimal coverage	• Target population: "harmful alcohol use" • "Coverage" defined as the proportion of harmful drinkers who actually receive BI • The paper also reported cost-effectiveness of treatment for alcohol dependence (data not shown here)
	Mortimer et al. (56)	2005	CUA: computer simulation	1) BI (variable 1-4 sessions; < 1 h total) vs. no BI 2) BI (5 minute session) vs. no BI 3) BI (20 minutes) vs. no BI 4) BI (120-150 minutes over 4 sessions) vs. no BI	1) $505 per QALY gained with BI 2) $62 per QALY gained with BI 3) $88 per QALY gained with BI 4) $213 per QALY gained with BI	• Target population: "problem drinkers" • Estimates for strategy 1 from Wilk et al. 1997 (2) • Estimates for strategies 2-4 from Saunders et al. 1991 (64) • Did not consider costs of screening or downstream cost-offsets from decreased alcohol-related health problems
	Dillie et al. (57)	2005	CBA: computer simulation	Screening with self-report plus CDT vs. self-report alone (positive screens received BI with 2 PCP visits and 2 follow-up phone calls)	Total cost savings of $212.30 for each patient screened with CDT	• Target population: primary care patients with hypertension and/or diabetes. Problem drinking defined as > 90 drinks/month for men and > 60 drinks/month for women • The comparison screening strategy (self-report) had a sensitivity of 40%, well below the sensitivity of recommended screening instruments (e.g., CAGE, AUDIT) • Outcome costs included medical costs,

TABLE 1 (continued)

Clinical Setting	Study	Year	Type of Analysis	Strategy Comparisons	Findings	Comments
Primary Care						
						motor vehicle accident costs, and legal costs from Project TrEAT (3,65)
	Babor et al. (48)	2006	Cost analysis: analysis within RCT	Practices randomized to 1) Usual care; 2) BI delivered by licensed practitioner (PCP, NP, PA); or 3) BI delivered by specialists (nurses)	Per-patient cost to deliver SBI was $4.87 in practitioner group and $3.53 in the specialist group	• Target population: primary care at-risk drinkers in managed care organizations • Costs collected prospectively • Details of cost analysis in Zarkin et al. 2003 (49)
Inpatient						
	Tolley et al. (58)	1991	CEA: analysis within observational study	Screening for at-risk drinking by doctors, nurses, and specialist workers	Compared to nurses, doctors cost $1.22 and specialist workers cost $1.95, respectively, to detect an additional case of at-risk drinking	• Target population: inpatients with at-risk drinking (> 36 units/week for men, > 24 units/week for women)
	Gentillelo et al. (59)	2005	CBA: computer simulation	SBI (30 minute BI) vs. no SBI	Savings of $3.81 for every $1.00 spent on SBI	• Target population: trauma patients with a blood alcohol level $\geq$ 100 mg/dL or a positive alcohol screening questionnaire • Analysis included patients discharged from emergency department
Emergency Department						
	Kunz et al. (60)	2004	CEA: analysis within RCT	BI vs. no BI	Compared to no BI, BI cost $2.45 to reduce AUDIT by 1 point, $2.89 to reduce alcohol use by 1 drink/week, and $10.34 to reduce the probability of heavy drinking by 1%	• Target population: at-risk drinkers in an inner-city ED • Preliminary findings per authors
	Barrett et al. (61)	2006	CEA: analysis within RCT	Information leaflet plus referral for BI (30-50 minutes) vs. information leaflet alone	Compared to leaflet alone, leaflet plus BI cost $32.03 per unit reduction in alcohol use per week	• Target population: hazardous drinkers (per Paddington Alcohol Test) presenting to ED • Only 33% of intervention group attended the BI

Abbreviations: AUDIT, Alcohol Use Disorders Identification Test; BI, brief intervention; CBA, cost-benefit analysis; CDT, carbohydrate deficient transferrin; CEA, cost-effectiveness analysis; CUA, cost-utility analysis; DALY, disability-adjusted life-year; ED, emergency department; ICER, incremental cost-effectiveness ratio; NP, nurse practitioner; QALY, quality-adjusted life-year; PA, physicians assistant; PCP, Primary Care Physician; RCT, randomized controlled trial; SBI, screening and brief intervention; USD, United States dollars; YLD, years lived with disability;

gram but not reporting health effects or benefits nor calculating an incremental ratio. Other summarized studies (50-61) are full economic evaluations (e.g., CBA, CEA, or CUA) that comprise a broad spectrum of data sources (literature review vs. prospective data collection), analytic technique (computer simulation and decision analytic models vs. standard statistical techniques), and assumptions. The remainder of this section describes some of the notable findings for each of the 3 medical settings.

Primary Care. Most studies summarized in Table 1 were conducted in primary care settings or, in the case of the computer simulations, were intended to influence primary care practice. Several population-based computer simulations (50,52,54,55,56) are categorized under primary care because they modeled BI delivered in primary care as one of their strategies. In a cost analysis of 212 primary care practices in the United Kingdom, Kaner et al. (47) found that 3 strategies (outreach training, training plus telephone support, and written guidelines) to encourage primary care nurses to perform alcohol SBI ranged in cost from $46.50 to $47.79 US dollars (USD) for each appropriate BI delivered. Conversely, in a US study of 15 primary care practices across 4 managed care organizations, Babor et al. (48) found an average incremental cost of $4.87 USD for each practitioner-delivered BI and $3.53 for each specialist (nurse)-delivered BI. The authors of both cost analyses concluded that SBI could be implemented and sustained in primary care at reasonable costs.

Several studies have used CBA to evaluate SBI in primary care. The most important are 2 studies from Fleming et al. (51,53) based on data from Project TrEAT (Trial for Early Alcohol Treatment), (3) a randomized controlled trial of BI for problem drinkers in primary care settings. At 12 months post-BI, the incremental benefit-cost ratio was 5.63:1 or a savings of $5.63 USD for every $1.00 USD spent on BI (51). At 48 months post-intervention, the ratio was 4.3:1 or a savings of $4.30 for every $1.00 spent on BI. (53) In a related study, Dillie et al. (57) used Project TrEAT and other data in a decision analytic CBA model to assess the new alcohol biomarker Carbohydrate Deficient Transferrin (CDT) as a screening tool for problem drinking in primary care. The analysis found a total cost savings of $212.30 USD for each patient screened with CDT. However, because the comparison screening strategy in this analysis was alcohol self-report with an estimated sensitivity of 40% for the detection of problem drinking, it is not known how the CDT strategy compares with the more sensitive alcohol screening questionnaires (e.g., CAGE, Alcohol Use Disorders Identification Test (AUDIT)) recommended in clinical guidelines.

The remaining primary care based studies in Table 1 used computer simulation to estimate the cost-effectiveness or cost-utility of SBI. Wutzke et al. (52) were one of the first to apply PHS Panel recommendations (7) to alcohol SBI. Using data from the Australian arm of the WHO BI Study Group, they found PCP-delivered BI (5 minutes) with minimal training support (defined in Table 1) cost $974 USD per life year saved when compared to usual care. In addition, a PCP-delivered BI with maximal training support cost $1492 USD per life year saved when compared to the BI with minimal support group. Although this study was limited by the absence of quality-of-life adjustment and some strong assumptions about mortality effects, it illustrated the application of CEA to evaluation of alcohol SBI programs. In a population-based CEA computer simulation, Andrews et al. (55) estimated the cost-effectiveness of BI at different coverage rates (defined as the proportion of harmful drinkers who actually receive BI). Compared to no BI, BI cost $6,593 USD and $10,250 USD per each year lived with disability averted when coverage was "current" at 8% and "optimal" at 70%, respectively.

To date, only 2 published economic evaluations of alcohol SBI in primary care have incorporated the utility measures necessary to conduct a CUA. As part of the WHO CHOICE (Choosing Interventions that are Cost Effective) program, (66) Chisholm et al. (54) found that, in Canada and the US, PCP-delivered BI cost $24,073 (in international dollars, a hypothetical unit of currency that reflects the worth of a country's currency within the country's borders) per DALY averted when compared to no BI. For this analysis, the hazardous drinking disability weight of 0.154 (where 0 = no disability and 1 = death) was derived from combination of Dutch disability weights for hazardous and harmful drinking (67). Likewise, Mortimer et al. (56) used the Dutch disability weights in a computer simulation CUA comparing BI of varying intensity for problem drinkers to no BI. Compared with no BI, the incremental cost per QALY ranged from $62 USD for a 5-minute BI to $505 USD for an aggregate BI [variable 1-4 sessions, total time < 1 hour, estimate from Wilk et al. (2)]. Additionally, preliminary findings from a decision-analytic, state-transition Markov model of alcohol SBI in primary care indicate lifetime cost savings of $300 and a gain of 0.05 QALYs for each patient screened (4,68).

Inpatient Settings. Despite the high prevalence of unhealthy alcohol use in the inpatient setting (69), only 2 economic evaluation studies of alcohol SBI for inpatients were found (Table 1). In a limited CEA within an observational study, Tolley et al. (58) found that, compared with nurses, doctors cost $1.22 USD and specialist workers cost $1.95 USD, respectively, to detect an additional case of at-risk drinking. In a computer simulation CBA, Gentillelo et al. (59) calculated a total savings of $3.81 USD for every $1.00 spent on SBI for trauma patients with a blood alcohol level ≥ 100 mg/dL and/or a positive alcohol screening questionnaire. No CUA studies with QALYs as the outcome were identified for inpatient alcohol SBI.

Emergency Department. Similar to the inpatient setting, only 2 economic evaluations of alcohol SBI were found for the ED (Table 1). Kunz et al. (60) conducted a preliminary CEA within a randomized controlled trial of BI for at-risk drinkers in an inner-city ED. Compared to no BI, BI cost $2.45 USD to reduce the AUDIT by 1 point, $2.89 USD to reduce alcohol use by 1 drink per week, and $10.34 USD to reduce the probability of heavy drinking by 1%. In a recent limited CEA targeted at hazardous drinkers presenting to an ED, Barrett et al. (61) found that provision of an information leaflet plus referral for a 30-minute BI cost $32.03 USD for each unit reduction in alcohol use per week when compared to provision of the leaflet only. This benefit occurred even though only 33% of the intervention group attended the BI session. No CUA studies with QALYs as the outcome were identified for inpatient alcohol SBI.

CONCLUSION

Despite the heterogeneity of methodological approaches, nearly all studies summarized in Table 1 support the use of alcohol SBI, particularly in the primary care setting. The full economic evaluations that prospectively collected cost and effect data (51,53) and conformed closely to methodological recommendations (51-54,59) strongly favored alcohol screening and brief intervention compared to usual care. Of these, the CBA studies showed cost benefits that were 3.8 to 5.6 times the cost of the SBI program whereas the CUA and CEA studies calculated cost per QALY or cost per life-year saved ratios that were well below external criterion thresholds considered to indicate "cost-effectiveness."

The other studies in Table 1 are more difficult to interpret. The studies which calculated the costs to implement and maintain a SBI program are useful within the context of program planning but do not indicate whether the health outcomes are "worth" the costs, especially when compared to programs competing for the same resources. Likewise, the studies which calculated the costs per clinical outcome (e.g., cost per problem drinker detected, cost per AUDIT score reduction, or cost per unit decrease in alcohol consumption) may be useful for direct comparison to other alcohol-directed programs but are not useful for general resource allocation decision-making because the health outcomes, unlike QALYs or DALYs, cannot be easily compared to outcomes of programs for non-alcohol related conditions.

The findings of the alcohol SBI economic evaluations discussed above have implications for both clinical care and future research. The highest quality primary care based studies in Table 1 indicate that alcohol SBI compares favorably to, and sometimes exceeds, the cost-effectiveness of many common primary care based preventive services, including aspirin prophylaxis, tobacco screening and intervention, colorectal cancer screening, influenza vaccination, pneumococcal vaccination, Chlamydia screening, and hypertension screening (70). Health care decision-makers and insurance payors can use these favorable comparative data as they consider the implementation of formal alcohol SBI programs in their primary care practices and the provision of financial coverage for alcohol SBI services, respectively.

Future research should focus on improving methods for measuring the costs and effects of alcohol SBI programs and for estimating the costs and effects over a longer period of time. Some specific research needs include, but are not limited to: (1) improved data on the effectiveness of alcohol SBI in "real world" settings, including non-primary care settings; (2) better estimates of short and long-term effects of alcohol use on clinical outcomes and quality of life; (3) more accurate utility estimates to allow calculation of QALYs and DALYs for a broader spectrum of unhealthy alcohol use and consequences; (4) a better understanding of how alcohol affects the quality of life of spouses and significant others; and (5) more sophisticated computer simulation models that track the complex natural history of healthy and unhealthy alcohol use, allow for repeated SBI over time, and are capable of state-of-the-art sensitivity analyses.

In summary, there has been significant progress in the application of economic evaluation to alcohol SBI in medical settings, with most studies indicating that such programs are a wise use of health care resources. There is ongoing methodological work to improve the estimation and measurement of costs and outcomes for the economic evaluation of alcohol and other substance abuse programs (12,26,71,72). As these methods improve, the estimates of the cost-effectiveness and cost-benefit of alcohol SBI programs should also improve and ensure accurate comparison to health care programs which compete for the same health care resources.

REFERENCES

1. Allen JP, Maisto SA, Connors GJ. Self-report screening tests for alcohol problems in primary care. Arch Int Med 1995;155:1726-1730.

2. Wilk AI, Jensen NM, Havighurst TC. Meta-analysis of randomized control trials addressing brief interventions in heavy alcohol drinkers. J Gen Int Med 1997;12:274-283.

3. Fleming MF, Barry KL, Manwell LB, Johnson K, London R. Brief physician advice for problem alcohol drinkers. A randomized controlled trial in community-based primary care practices. JAMA 1997;277: 1039-1045.

4. Saitz R, Svikis D, D'Onofrio G, Kraemer KL, Perl H. Challenges applying alcohol brief intervention in diverse practice settings: populations, outcomes, and costs. Alcohol Clin Exp Res 2006;30:332-338.

5. Saitz R. Clinical practice: Unhealthy alcohol use. N Engl J Med 2005;352:596-607.

6. McLellan AT. Technology transfer and the treatment of addiction: what can research offer practice? J Subst Abuse Treatment 2002;22:169-170.

7. Gold MR, Russell LB, Seigel JE, Weinstein MC, eds. *Cost-effectiveness in health and medicine*. New York: Oxford University Press; 1996.

8. Drummond MF, Sculpher M, Stoddart GL, O'Brien BJ, Torrance GW. *Methods for the economic evaluation of health care programmes*. 3rd ed. Oxford: Oxford University Press; 2005.

9. Weinstein M, Stason W. Foundations of cost-effectiveness analysis for health and medical practices. N Eng J Med 1977;13:716-721.

10. Detsky AS, Naglie G. A clinician's guide to cost-effectiveness analysis. Ann Intern Med 1990;113: 147-154.

11. Zarkin GA, French MT, Anderson DW, Bradley CJ. A conceptual framework for the economic evaluation of substance abuse interventions. Evaluation and Program Planning 1994;17:409-418.

12. Bray JW, Zarkin GA. Economic evaluation of alcoholism treatment. Alcohol Res Health 2006;29:27-33.

13. French MT. Economic evaluation of alcohol treatment services. Recent Developments in Alcoholism 2001;15:209-228.

14. Holder HD, Hallan JB. Impact of alcoholism treatment on total health care costs: a six-year study. Advances in Alcohol & Substance Abuse 1986;6:1-15.

15. Holder HD, Shachtman RH. Estimating health care savings associated with alcoholism treatment. Alcohol Clin Exp Res 1987;11:66-73.

16. Holder HD, Blose JO. The reduction of health care costs associated with alcoholism treatment: a 14-year longitudinal study. J Stud Alcohol 1992;53: 293-302.

17. Jones KR, Vischi TR. Impact of alcohol, drug abuse and mental health treatment on medical care utilization. A review of the research literature. Med Care 1979;17(Suppl 2):1-82.

18. Hunkeler EM, Hung YY, Rice DP, Weisner C, Hu T. Alcohol consumption patterns and health care costs in an HMO. Drug Alcohol Depend 2001;64: 181-190.

19. Hayashida M, Alterman AI, McLellan AT, et al. Comparative effectiveness and costs of inpatient and outpatient detoxification of patients with mild-to-moderate alcohol withdrawal syndrome. N Eng J Med 1989;320:358-365.

20. McKenna M, Chick J, Buxton M, Howlett H, Patience D, Ritson B. The SECCAT survey: I. The costs

and consequences of alcoholism. Alcohol Alcohol 1996;31:565-576.

21. Weisner C, Mertens J, Parthasarathy S, Moore C, Lu Y. Integrating primary medical care with addiction treatment: a randomized controlled trial. JAMA 2001;286:1715-1723.

22. Weisner C, Mertens J, Parthasarathy S, et al. The outcome and cost of alcohol and drug treatment in an HMO: day hospital versus traditional outpatient regimens. Health Services Res 2000;35:791-812.

23. Cisler R, Holder HD, Longabaugh R, Stout RL, Zweben A. Actual and estimated replication costs for alcohol treatment modalities: case study from Project MATCH. J Stud Alcohol 1998;59:503-512.

24. Holder HD, Cisler RA, Longabaugh R, Stout RL, Treno AJ, Zweben A. Alcoholism treatment and medical care costs from Project MATCH. Addiction 2000; 95:999-1013.

25. Mishan EJ. *Cost-benefit analysis*. London, UK: Allen and Unwin; 1971.

26. French MT, Salome HJ, Sindelar JL, McLellan AT. Benefit-cost analysis of addiction treatment: methodological guidelines and empirical application using the DATCAP and ASI. Health Services Res 2002; 37:433-455.

27. Cartwright WS. Cost-benefit analysis of drug treatment services: review of the literature. J Ment Health Policy Econ 2000;3:11-26.

28. Zarkin GA, Hubbard RL. Analytic issues for estimating the benefits and costs of substance abuse prevention. NIDA Research Monographs. 1998;(Monograph No.176):141-160.

29. Sindelar JL, Manning WG. Cost-benefit and cost-effectiveness analysis: Issues in the evalulation of the treatment of illicit drug abuse. In: Egertson J, Fox D, Leshner A, eds. *Treating Drug Abusers Effectively*. London: Milbank/Blackwell; 1997:187-222.

30. Hubbard RL, French MT. New perspectives on the benefit-cost and cost-effectiveness of drug abuse treatment. In: Kaple JM, ed. *Economic Costs, Cost-Effectiveness, Financing, and Community-Based Drug Treatment, Research Monograph No. 113, DHHS Publication No. ADM 91-1823*. Rockville, MD: National Institute on Drug Abuse; 1991:94-113.

31. Tsevat J, Weeks JC, Guadagnoli E, et al. Using health-related quality-of-life information: clinical encounters, clinical trials, and health policy. J Gen Intern Med 1994;9:576-582.

32. Patrick D, Erickson P. *Health status and health policy: Quality of life in health care evaluation and resource allocation*. New York: Oxford University Press; 1993.

33. Torrance GW, Feeny D. Utilities and quality-adjusted life years. Int J Tech Assess Health Care 1989;5:559-575.

34.Chapman RH, Stone PW, Sandberg EA, Bell C, Neumann PJ. A comprehensive league table of cost-utility ratios and a sub-table of "panel-worthy" studies. Med Decision Making 2000;20:451-467.

35. Goldman L, Phillips KA, Coxson P, et al. The effect of risk factor reductions between 1981 and 1990 on coronary heart disease incidence, prevalence, mortality and cost. J American College Cardio 2001;38: 1012-1017.

36. Phillips KA, Shlipak MG, Coxson P, et al. Health and economic benefits of increased beta-blocker use following myocardial infarction. JAMA 2000;284: 2748-2754.

37. Tosteson AN, Weinstein MC, Hunink MG, et al. Cost-effectiveness of population wide educational approaches to reduce serum cholesterol levels. Circ 1997;95:24-30.

38. Matchar DB, Samsa GP, Matthews JR, et al. The Stroke Prevention Policy Model: linking evidence and clinical decisions. Ann Intern Med 1997;127:704-711.

39. Freedberg KA, Losina E, Weinstein MC, et al. The cost effectiveness of combination antiretroviral therapy for HIV disease. N Eng J Med 2001;344: 824-831.

40. Towse A, Pritchard C. National Institute for Clinical Excellence (NICE): Is economic appraisal working? Pharmacoeconomics 2002;20 (Suppl 3):95-105.

41. Gafni A, Birch S. NICE methodological guidelines and decision making in the National Health Service in England and Wales. Pharmacoeconomics 2003; 21:149-157.

42. Glennie JL, Torrance GW, Baladi JF, et al. The revised Canadian Guidelines for the economic evaluation of pharmaceuticals. Pharmacoeconomics 1999;15: 459-468.

43. Hirth RA, Chernew ME, Miller E, Fendrick AM, Weissert WG. Willingness to pay for a quality-adjusted life year: in search of a standard. Med Decision Making 2000;20:332-342.

44. Ubel PA, Hirth RA, Chernew ME, Fendrick AM. What is the price of life and why doesn't it increase at the rate of inflation? Arch Intern Med 2003;163: 1637-1641.

45. Sindelar JL, Jofre-Bonet M, French MT, McLellan AT. Cost-effectiveness analysis of addiction treatment: paradoxes of multiple outcomes. Drug Alcohol Depend 2004;73:41-50.

46. Weinstein M, Manning W. Theoretical issues in cost-effectiveness analysis. J Health Econ 1997;16: 121-128.

47. Kaner E, Lock C, Heather N, McNamee P, Bond S. Promoting brief alcohol intervention by nurses in primary care: a cluster randomised controlled trial. Patient Education & Counseling 2003;51:277-284.

48. Babor TF, Higgins-Biddle JC, Dauser D, Burleson JA, Zarkin GA, Bray J. Brief interventions for at-risk drinking: patient outcomes and cost-effectiveness in managed care organizations. Alcohol Alcohol 2006;41: 624-631.

49. Zarkin GA, Bray JW, Davis KL, Babor TF, Higgins-Biddle JC. The costs of screening and brief intervention for risky alcohol use. J Stud Alcohol 2003; 64:849-857.

50. Lindholm L. Alcohol advice in primary health care–is it a wise use of resources? Health Policy 1998;45:47-56.

51. Fleming MF, Mundt MP, French MT, Manwell LB, Stauffacher EA, Barry KL. Benefit-cost analysis of brief physician advice with problem drinkers in primary care settings. Med Care 2000;38:7-18.

52. Wutzke SE, Shiell A, Gomel MK, Conigrave KM. Cost effectiveness of brief interventions for reducing alcohol consumption. Soc Science Med 2001;52: 863-870.

53. Fleming MF, Mundt MP, French MT, Manwell LB, Stauffacher EA, Barry KL. Brief physician advice for problem drinkers: long-term efficacy and benefit-cost analysis. Alcohol Clin Exp Res 2002;26:36-43.

54. Chisholm D, Rehm J, Van Ommeren M, Monteiro M. Reducing the global burden of hazardous alcohol use: a comparative cost-effectiveness analysis. J Stud Alcohol 2004;65:782-793.

55. Andrews G, Issakidis C, Sanderson K, et al. Utilising survey data to inform public policy: comparison of the cost-effectiveness of treatment of ten mental disorders. Br J Psychiatry 2004;184: 526-533.

56. Mortimer D, Segal L. Economic evaluation of interventions for problem drinking and alcohol dependence: cost per QALY estimates. Alcohol Alcohol 2005; 40:549-555.

57. Dillie KS, Mundt M, French MT, et al. Cost-benefit analysis of a new alcohol biomarker, Carbohydrate Deficient Transferrin, in a chronic illness primary care sample. Alcohol Clin Exp Res 2005;29:2008-2014.

58. Tolley K, Rowland N. Identification of alcohol-related problems in a general hospital setting: a cost-effectiveness evaluation. Br J Addict 1991;86: 429-438.

59. Gentilello LM, Ebel BE, Wickizer TM, Salkever DS, Rivara FP. Alcohol interventions for trauma patients treated in emergency departments and hospitals: a cost benefit analysis. Ann Surg 2005;241:541-550.

60. Kunz FM Jr, French MT, Bazargan-Hejazi S. Cost-effectiveness analysis of a brief intervention delivered to problem drinkers presenting at an inner-city hospital emergency department. J Stud Alcohol 2004; 65:363-370.

61. Barrett B, Byford S, Crawford MJ, Patton R, Drummond C, Henry JA, Touquet R. Cost-effectiveness of screening and referral to an alcohol health worker in alcohol misusing patients attending an accident and emergency department: a decision-making approach. Drug Alcohol Depend 2006;81:47-54.

62. King MB. Case finding for at risk drinking in general practice: cost-benefit analysis. Psychological Medicine 1986;16:359-363.

63. Gomel MK, Wutzke SE, Hardcastle DM, Lapsley H, Reznik RB. Cost-effectiveness of strategies to market and train primary health care physicians in brief intervention techniques for hazardous alcohol use. Soc Sci Med 1998; 47:203-211.

64. Saunders JB, Hanratty SJ, Burns RH, et al. Successful early intervention for harmful alcohol consumption: results from the WHO randomized controlled trial. Proceedings of the Autumn School for Studies in Alcohol and Drugs 1991; 183-192.

65. Mundt MP. Analyzing the costs and benefits of brief intervention. Alcohol Research and Health 2006; 29:34-35.

66. World Health Organization. WHO-CHOICE Cost-effectiveness analyses. Geneva: World Health Organization, 2004. http://www.who.int/whosis

67. Stouthard ME, Essink-Bot ML, Bonsel GL on behalf of the Dutch Disability Weights Group. Disability weights for diseases: a modified protocol and results for a Western European region. Europ J Publ Hlth 2000;10:24-30.

68. Kraemer KL, Roberts MS, Freedner N, Palfai T, Saitz R. Cost-effectiveness of alcohol screening in primary care: applying national recommendations for cost-effectiveness analysis to alcohol use disorders. Alcohol Clin Exp Res 2004;28(suppl):164A.

69. Saitz R, Freedner N, Palfai TP, Horton NJ, Samet JH. The severity of unhealthy alcohol use in hospitalized medical patients: the spectrum is narrow. J Gen Intern Med 2006;21:381-385.

70. Maciosek MV, Coffield AB, Edwards NM, Flottemesch TJ, Goodman MJ, Solberg LI. Priorities among effective clinical preventive services: results of a systematic review and analysis. Am J Prev Med 2006; 31:52-61.

71. Kraemer KL, Roberts MS, Horton NJ, Palfai T, Samet JH, Freedner N, Tibbetts N, Saitz R. Health utility ratings for a spectrum of alcohol-related health states. Medical Care 2005;43:541-550.

72. Jofre-Bonet M, Sindelar JL. Creating an aggregate outcome index: cost-effectiveness analysis of substance abuse treatment. J Behav Health Services Research 2004;31:229-241.

doi:10.1300/J465v28n03_07

An Evidence-Based Alcohol Screening, Brief Intervention and Referral to Treatment (SBIRT) Curriculum for Emergency Department (ED) Providers Improves Skills and Utilization

The Academic ED SBIRT Research Collaborative

SUMMARY. *Objective:* Emergency Departments (EDs) offer an opportunity to improve the care of patients with at-risk and dependent drinking by teaching staff to screen, perform brief interven-

Presented at the Society of Academic Emergency Medicine (SAEM) Annual Meeting, May 2005.
Presented at the Research Society on Alcoholism (RSA) Meeting, June 2005.
Address correspondence to: Edward Bernstein, MD, Professor and Vice-Chair for Academic Affairs, Department of Emergency Medicine, Boston University School of Medicine, One Boston Medical Center Place, Boston MA 02118 (E-mail: ebernste@bu.edu).
Funded in part by NIAAA 1R25AA014957, 1R03AA01511-14.
There are no financial arrangements that represent conflict of interest.
Collaborative authors include (in alphabetical order): BOSTON UNIVERSITY: Edward Bernstein, MD, Judith Bernstein, RNC, PhD, James Feldman, MD, William Fernandez, MD, Melissa Hagan, MPH, Patricia Mitchell, RN, Clara Safi, RNP; BROWN UNIVERSITY: Robert Woolard, MD, Mike Mello, MD, Janette Baird, PhD, Cristina Lee, PhD; CHARLES R. DREW UNIVERSITY: Shahrzad Bazargan-Hejazi, PhD; DENVER HEALTH MEDICAL CENTER: Kerry Broderick, MD, Kathryn A. LaPerrier, CSW; EMORY UNIVERSITY: Arthur Kellermann, MD, MPH, Marlena M. Wald, MLS, MPH; HOWARD UNIVERSITY: Robert E. Taylor, MD, PhD, Kim Walton, PhD, Michelle Grant-Ervin, MD; TUFTS UNIVERSITY: Denise Rollinson, MD, David Edwards; UNIVERSITY OF CALIFORNIA, SAN DIEGO: Theodore Chan, MD, Dan Davis, MD, Jean Buchanan Marshall, MS, RN; UNIVERSITY OF CONNECTICUT HEALTH CENTER: Robert Aseltine, Jr., PhD, Amy James, PhD; Elizabeth Schilling, PhD; Khamis Abu-Hasaballah, PhD; UNIVERSITY OF MEDICINE AND DENTISTRY OF NEW JERSEY ROBERT WOOD JOHNSON MEDICAL SCHOOL AT CAMDEN: Brigitte M. Baumann, MD, Edwin D. Boudreaux, PhD; UNIVERSITY OF MICHIGAN: Ronald Maio, DO, MS, Rebecca Cunningham, MD, Teresa Murrell, RN, CCRC; UNIVERSITY OF NEW MEXICO: David Doezema, MD, Michael J. Bauer, BA; UNIVERSITY OF SOUTHERN CALIFORNIA: Deirdre Anglin, MD, MPH, Adriana Eliassen, RN; UNIVERSITY OF VIRGINIA: Marcus Martin, MD, Jesse Pines, MD, Leslie Buchanan, NP, James Turner, MD; YALE UNIVERSITY: Gail D'Onofrio, MD, Linda C. Degutis, DrPH, Patricia Owens, MS.

[Haworth co-indexing entry note]: "An Evidence-Based Alcohol Screening, Brief Intervention and Referral to Treatment (SBIRT) Curriculum for Emergency Department (ED) Providers Improves Skills and Utilization." The Academic ED SBIRT Research Collaborative. Co-published simultaneously in *Substance Abuse* (The Haworth Medical Press, an imprint of The Haworth Press, Inc.) Vol. 28, No. 4, 2007, pp. 79-92; and: *Alcohol/Drug Screening and Brief Intervention: Advances in Evidence-Based Practice* (ed: Richard Saitz, and Marc Galanter) The Haworth Medical Press, an imprint of The Haworth Press, Inc., 2007, pp. 79-92. Single or multiple copies of this article are available for a fee from The Haworth Document Delivery Service [1-800-HAWORTH, 9:00 a.m. - 5:00 p.m. (EST). E-mail address: docdelivery@haworthpress.com].

Available online at http://suba.haworthpress.com

doi:10.1300/J465v28n04_01

tion and refer to treatment (SBIRT). We describe here the implementation at 14 Academic EDs of a structured SBIRT curriculum to determine if this learning experience improves provider beliefs and practices.

Methods: ED faculty, residents, nurses, physician extenders, social workers, and Emergency Medical Technicians (EMTs) were surveyed prior to participating in either a two hour interactive workshops with case simulations, or a web-based program (www.ed.bmc.org/sbirt). A pre-post repeated measures design assessed changes in provider beliefs and practices at three and 12 months post-exposure.

Results: Among 402 ED providers, 74% reported < 10 hours of prior professional alcohol-related education and 78% had < 2 hours exposure in the previous year. At 3-month follow-up, scores for self-reported confidence in ability, responsibility to intervene, and actual utilization of SBIRT skills all improved significantly over baseline. Gains decreased somewhat at 12 months, but remained above baseline. Length of time in practice was positively associated with SBIRT utilization, controlling for gender, race and type of profession. Persistent barriers included time limitations and lack of referral resources.

Conclusions: ED providers respond favorably to SBIRT. Changes in utilization were substantial at three months post-exposure to a standardized curriculum, but less apparent after 12 months. Booster sessions, trained assistants and infrastructure supports may be needed to sustain changes over the longer term. doi:10.1300/J465v28n04_01

KEYWORDS. Brief intervention, alcohol screening, substance abuse, alcohol education

INTRODUCTION

The Rationale for Emergency Department (ED) Screening

The estimated cost of alcohol abuse and dependence for health care, lost productivity, property damage, criminal justice system involvement and loss of life in the US is in excess of $185 billion.[1] In 2001-2002, the 12 month prevalence for alcohol abuse or dependence was 17.6 million or 8.5% of the U.S. population, and 29.3% of the population exceeded recommended drinking limits.[2] There were approximately 75,000 alcohol attributable deaths associated with 2.3 million years of potential life lost,[3] with half of these deaths attributed to binge drinking (consumption of 5 or more drinks for men and 4 or more drinks for women in a 2 hour occasion).[4] Binge drinking also resulted in 14,600 motor vehicle crash deaths and increased the risk of injury nine-fold.

Furthermore, out of 110 million ED visits in 2001, 7.6 million were attributable to alcohol.[5] ED patients are 1.5-3.0 times more likely to report heavy drinking or consequences than those in primary care.[6] Among ED patients, 31% screen positive on the CAGE instrument (≥ 2 questions),[7] more than 10% of patients meet DSM-IV or ICD-10 criteria for alcohol dependence,[8] and 25% are positive on the Alcohol Use Disorders Identification Test (AUDIT) using a probability sample.[9] In a five year follow-up, alcohol intoxicated ED patients had twice the mortality rate as the non-intoxicated comparison group.[10]

Current rates of screening in the ED are inadequate to identify and address alcohol problems, and alcohol on breath is insufficient as a diagnostic procedure.[7] If 10% of ED patients meet criteria for dependence and another 20% meet criteria for possible dependence with CAGE >2, then one might estimate conservatively that at least 10 million ED visits in any given year should be associated with a referral for assessment and/or treatment contact, and many millions of high risk drinkers, who are not dependent but simply drinking at levels that have negative health effects, would benefit from brief intervention. In 2001, however, only 11.4% of the 2.5 million patients whose visit was directly related to alcohol use (those with an alcohol attributable medical condition) were referred for treatment.[11,12] These findings provide compelling clinical and public health reasons for the ED to institute systems for alcohol screening, brief intervention and referral to treatment (SBIRT) in order to improve the care of patients with high risk or dependent drinking.

The Potential for Brief Intervention in the ED

SBIRT has been tested for over 20 years in primary care/general medicine settings. A systematic review of randomized controlled trials by the US Preventive Service Task Force found that at least one 15 minute conversation by a primary care provider resulted in 2.9-8.7 fewer mean drinks per week (13%-34% net reduction) and a 10%-19% increase in the number of persons drinking at moderate to safe levels, compared to control groups.[13] Some early ED studies support this use of brief intervention to reduce high risk drinking and associated consequences. For example, in a trial of a 40 minute motivational intervention plus follow-up booster by non ED providers, investigators at Brown Medical School reported that sub-critically injured drinking patients in the intervention group had fewer alcohol-related injuries and consequences than controls at 12 month follow-up. In the subgroup of patients presenting as a result of motor vehicle crashes, the intervention group had 1/3 fewer alcohol related injuries than controls.[14,15]

In a systematic review of four ED based studies of brief intervention, D'Onofrio and Degutis conclude that ED intervention is effective, and recommend that ED screening and brief intervention be incorporated into clinical practice.[16] While it is not yet clear which subgroups of ED patients are most likely to benefit,[17] there is clearly a need to evaluate SBIRT in the ED setting. Here we report results from the implementation of a standardized SBIRT curriculum for ED providers that was designed as part of a 14 site trial of SBIRT with ED patients who screen positive for high risk or dependent drinking.

Implementation of a Standardized Curriculum in a Single ED Site

In 1998, D'Onofrio et al. conducted a small controlled trial of a structured educational intervention for ED residents (n = 36) at two sites using a pre-post survey, and demonstrated improvement in knowledge scores and increase in documentation of screening and intervention from 17% to 58% on the medical charts reviewed.[18] Building on this earlier work, D'Onofrio and colleagues at Yale then developed and successfully implemented an innovative skills-based educational program for a variety of emergency practitioners.[19] ED faculty, residents and physicians' assistants demonstrated their proficiency in a brief negotiation interview, the BNI, using standardized patient scenarios. During the 2002-2003 study period, 47 ED providers performed a total of 247 interventions with a mean duration time of 7.75 minutes. This study demonstrated the need to test a standardized curriculum with a wider population of ED practitioners, and set the stage for a multi-centered trial of a standardized SBIRT curriculum.

Translation to Academic EDs Across the Nation

In March 2003, the Society for Academic Emergency Medicine (SAEM) and the National Institute on Alcohol Abuse and Alcoholism (NIAAA) invited the National Alcohol Screening Day (NASD) working group to help develop a translational research study to determine whether ED providers can implement SBIRT under real-time ED conditions and link provider performance to improvements in ED patient outcomes.

Academic Emergency Departments were selected as a focus for this dissemination effort because this setting offered a conjunction of *need* (high problem prevalence but no alcohol content in the ED training curriculum other than acute clinical care) and *opportunity* (the availability of an existing structure of weekly conferences for resident education). This familiar venue was critical to acceptance of SBIRT training, because (1) physicians and nurses were being asked to step outside their content comfort zone of pathophysiology of alcohol to focus on communication skills for behavior change, an area of less expertise, and (2) to step outside the ED paradigm of crisis care to learn skills aimed at prevention (for the high risk drinker) or treatment of chronic conditions (for the dependent drinker). Because didactic approaches to altering medical practice have not proved to be very successful,[19] we selected a more effective strategy of interactive, skills-based format.[20]

Syllabi and educational materials developed for the primary care setting are not readily accepted by emergency physicians, because the conditions of practice–acuity, time constraints, patient management by a multidisciplinary team, delegation of duties, planned discontinuity of care, legally mandated, uncontrolled access, and crisis-oriented scope of mission–are so different from those that obtain in the usual physician-patient relationship. A psychiatrist might define brief intervention as 10 sessions, a primary care provider might define it as three short visits, but for the ED staff, the window of opportunity for brief intervention might be only 10 minutes, with the baton then passed to someone else. We describe here the evidence-based SBIRT curriculum that was therefore designed specifically for ED providers, its implementation at 14 academic ED sites, and its impact on the practices and beliefs of ED physicians, nurses (RNs), nurse practitioners (NPs), physicians' assistants (PAs), social workers and Emergency Medical Technicians (EMTs).

METHODS

Study Design

This trial of an educational intervention was embedded within a controlled comparison of the effect of SBIRT on ED patient outcomes at 14 sites. Institutional Review Board approval for the provider component was obtained at each of the fourteen sites, and at the Alcohol Education Project parent site at Boston University, and written informed consent was obtained from all participating providers. A pre-post-retention repeated measures design was used to test the hypothesis that ED providers from a variety of disciplines would change their beliefs and practices at 3 and 12 months post exposure to a standardized SBIRT curriculum. In *Phase I*, the control period in Spring, 2004, 40 ED patients at each site who screened positive for high risk or dependent drinking were enrolled by a study coordinator or designated research assistant. In *Phase II*, ED providers enrolled in the study, completed a pretest about alcohol beliefs and professional experiences and practices, and were exposed to the SBIRT curriculum via local workshop or via web-based learning module. In *Phase III* (Late Spring and Early Summer, 2004), the enrolled ED providers had the opportunity to participate in a trial of screening, brief intervention and referral of ED patients at each site during their clinical shifts. In *Phase IV*, ED providers completed a post-test at 3 months and 12 months.

Sample

During the spring of 2004, each of the 14 sites issued an invitation to ED faculty, residents, nurses, nurse practitioners, physician's assistants, social workers, EMTs and other ED based staff to enroll in the study.

Setting

The 14 academic ED sites participating in the study were affiliated with the following institutions: Boston University, Brown University, Charles R. Drew University, Denver Health Medical Center, Emory University, Howard University, Tufts University, University of California San Diego, University of Medicine and Dentistry of New Jersey, University of Michigan, University of New Mexico, University of Southern California (LAC), University of Virginia and Yale University. These urban and suburban teaching hospitals with ED residency programs, who represented all regions of the country and served a large, diverse patient population, each received an RO3 from NIAAA to fund their participation in the study.

Curriculum Components

The curriculum consisted of: (1) a 30 minute slide show on the rationale for and research supporting SBIRT effectiveness; (2) a series of five video cases in which ED providers demonstrate intervention skills and the BNI algorithm with simulated patients; (3) scripted scenarios for practicing skills; (4) pocket sized plastic cards with NIAAA screening guidelines, a graphic display of typical drinks and the intervention algorithm; and (5) a web site designed for independent learning (www.ed.bmc.org/sbirt).

A research team and an educational coordinator at each site facilitated all aspects of the program including assisting practitioners with independent learning. Boston University and Yale University provided technical assistance, curriculum development and instructors for local workshops at each site.

Curriculum Content

The Two Minute Screen

The screening protocol consisted of three questions prefaced by the statement, "I ask all my patients these questions in order to give better care. Would you mind answering them?"

- On average, how many days per week do you drink alcohol (beer, wine, liquor)?
- On a typical day when you drink, how many drinks do you have?
- What is the maximum number of drinks you had on any given occasion during the last month?

A standard drink is defined as 12 ounces of beer, 6 ounces of wine or 1.5 ounces of liquor. National Institute of Alcohol Abuse and Alcoholism epidemiologically based guidelines for low risk consumption [22] were taught to providers. According to these guidelines, drinking at the following levels puts patients at risk for injury or illness and constitutes a positive screen:

- >14 drinks/week for men
- >7 drinks/week for women
- >1 drink per day for those 65 years or older
- > 0 drinks during pregnancy and for those dependent on alcohol or on medications that interact with alcohol
- > 4 drinks for men and >3 drinks for women per 2 hour drinking occasion

Development of the BNI Intervention

The intervention, a discussion designed to be completed in 5-10 minutes, is built on best practices derived from the literature.[23-27] The goal of the brief intervention curriculum was to offer ED providers an array of skills/tools that can be adapted to any particular situation they encounter in interacting with patients with high risk or dependent drinking, since resistance to discussion of behavior change is normally expected. The BNI was designed to be efficient, effective, respectful, and satisfying to both patient and practitioner, and give patients a voice and a choice. The original version was developed in 1994 for Project ASSERT at the Boston Medical Center ED with the help of Dr. Stephen Rollnick,[28] and is illustrated in the video, "The Emergency Physician and the Problem Drinker."[29] D'Onofrio, Pantalon et al. further adapted and standardized the intervention as an algorithm for Project ED Health, 2001.[19] These two versions were merged for the current study.

Key Elements of the BNI

After asking permission to raise the subject, the ED provider reviews screening results in light of the NIAAA guidelines for low risk drinking, and assists the patient to make a connection between alcohol use and the reason for visit or stated health concerns (Figure 1). The provider then works with the patient to enhance motivation, developing discrepancies between the benefits and losses that the patient associates with drinking and between the patient's current life situation and his/her future goals. The patient's natural resistance to change can be mitigated by avoiding judgmental labeling and finger pointing, through reflective listening based on empathy and respect, and by building on previous attempts at change. The readiness ruler with which a patient identifies his or her level of readiness to change (on a scale of 1 to 10) offers a technique to help patients to voice their own concerns. The provider's question "why not a lower number" may elicit change talk such as, "I crashed my car tonight, cut up my face and spent six hours in the ER getting sutured and X-rayed, so I've got to slow down a bit." The provider reinforces positive commitment statements, because the number of such statements and their salience is associated with positive change and better outcomes.[30] The next step is to negotiate a specific action plan (prescription for change) with the patient to reduce risks and consequences related to drinking. The semi-structured format is the method cited as most closely associated with better effect size and outcomes.[31]

FIGURE 1. SBIRT Algorithm as Taught in the Standardized ED Curriculum

BNI STEPS	DIALOGUE/PROCEDURES
1. Raise subject	➢ Hello, I am _______. Would you mind taking a few minutes to talk with me about your alcohol use? **<<PAUSE and LISTEN>>**
2. Provide feedback	
• **Review screen**	➢ From what I understand you are drinking [insert screening data]... We know that drinking above certain levels can cause problems, such as [insert facts]...I am concerned about your drinking.
• **Make connection**	➢ What connection (if any) do you see between your drinking and this ED visit? **If patient sees connection:** reiterate what pt has said **If patient does not see connection:** make one using facts
• **Show NIAAA guidelines & norms**	➢ These are what we consider the upper limits of low risk drinking for your age and sex. By low risk we mean that you would be less likely to experience illness or injury if you stayed within these guidelines.
3. Enhance motivation	
• **Readiness to change**	➢ **[Show readiness ruler]** On a scale from 1-10, how ready are you to change any aspect of your drinking?
• **Develop discrepancy**	➢ **If patient says:** **≥2 ask** Why did you choose that number and not a lower one?
• **Explore Pros and Cons**	**≤3 or resistance ask pros and cons** Help me to understand what you enjoy about drinking? **<<PAUSE AND LISTEN>>** Now tell me what you enjoy less about drinking. **<<PAUSE AND LISTEN>>**
• **Use Reflective Listening**	➢ On the one hand you said, **<<RESTATE PROS>>** ➢ On the other hand you said, **<<RESTATE CONS>>** So tell me, where does this leave you?
4. Negotiate & advise	
• **Negotiate goal**	➢ What's the next step?
• **Give advice**	➢ What do you think you can do to stay within the safe drinking guidelines? If you can stay within these limits you will be less likely to experience [further] illness or injury related to alcohol use.
• **Summarize**	➢ This is what I've heard you say...Here is a drinking agreement I would like you to fill out, reinforcing your new drinking goals. This is really an agreement between you and yourself. Provide drinking agreement [patient keeps 1 copy]
• **Provide handouts and suggest PC f/u**	➢ **Suggest Primary Care follow-up to discuss drinking level/pattern**
• **Thank patient**	➢ **Thank patient for his/her time**

ED=Emergency Department; BNI=Brief Negotiated Interview; SBIRT=Screening, Brief Intervention and Referral to Treatment; PC=Primary care; NIAAA=National Institute of Alcohol Abuse and Alcoholism

Adapted from 19,28,29

Referral Resources

Each site was assisted to develop a resource/referral list and to work closely with social workers, addiction counselors, and Alcoholics Anonymous volunteers, and to use the Center for Substance Abuse Treatment's Treatment finder web site.[32] Patients are encouraged to take responsibility for lifestyle change, explore personal and community resources for change, and make decisions that they think they can actually carry out.

Measurement

An *ED Clinician Survey* adapted from D'Onofrio et al.[18] was administered prior to SBIRT exposure and at 3 and 12 months post training. The survey includes demographics, prior exposure to an alcohol curriculum, beliefs about alcohol and about intervention, and an inventory of current practices with patients who are high risk or dependent drinkers. Likert-format survey responses (scale:1-5) at baseline and at follow-up were compared for changes in the following domains: (1) perceived ability to conduct SBIRT skills, (2) responsibility to conduct SBIRT, (3) perceived barriers, and (4) self reported utilization of SBIRT skills. Composite mean scores were calculated from the responses to the screening, brief intervention and referral questions within each domain. For example, in the utilization domain, the following questions were asked [never to always]:

- How often do you ask patients about their alcohol problems?
- How often do you ask about quantity and frequency of use?
- How often do you formally screen patients using CAGE?
- How often do you assess patients' readiness to change?
- How often do you discuss/advise patients to change their drinking behavior?
- How often do you refer patients with alcohol problems?
- How often do you document your assessment, intervention and referral?

For responsibility, the question was phrased as, "What do you think is your responsibility as an emergency physician, nurse or physicians' assistant to do the following [same items, no responsibility to major responsibility]?" For confidence, the questions were phrased as "Rate the following statements according to your confidence/ability level [from no confidence to high confidence]. I am confident in my ability to . . . [same items]."

Data Analysis

Chi-square analysis was used for bivariate comparison of nominal data. Paired *t* tests were performed for pre-post comparison of composite mean scores, and an OLS regression model was developed for analysis of independent predictors. SPSS® software was used for analysis.

RESULTS

Participants

The 402 ED providers were enrolled; 83% (n = 334) were reassessed at 3 months, and 72% (n = 288) were reassessed at 12 months.

Baseline Survey

Participants were 52% male, and diverse in their disciplines (60% MDs, 21% RNs, 7% RNP or PAs, and 8% social workers and 3% EMTs). Among the physicians, 31% were residents, and there was variation of length of time in practice from 1-5 years (14%) to 6-10 years (16%) to 10 + years (38%). The majority (74%) attended workshops; the remainder used the website for independent learning or small group sessions.

Previous alcohol related training and experience: While 68% rated their past experience working with patients with alcohol problems as 'moderate' or 'large,' 74% reported having less than 10 hours of alcohol education during graduate or post-graduate training, and 78% reported less than 2 hours of alcohol education in the previous year.

Pre-Post Comparisons at 3 Months

Providers who completed the three month follow-up survey were not different in demographics, alcohol experience or training or alcohol beliefs from those who were lost to follow-up. Paired samples *t*-tests demonstrated improvement post-exposure to the SBIRT curriculum in all four domains (see Table 1).

Skills and responsibility at 3 months: Confidence in ability to perform SBIRT skills improved by 11%, and perception of responsibility to provide SBIRT increased by 7%.

Barriers to SBIRT utilization at 3 months: Items assessed included lack of time, lack of referral resources, legal issues about documentation, lack of role models among faculty for screening, potential for angry response from patients, and lack of belief in effectiveness of treatment. At post-test, barriers were rated as less troublesome but by a decrease of only 3%. Overall, providers indicated a greater belief that SBIRT would make a difference (mean score 3.65 at baseline vs. 3.93 at 3 months, a difference of 0.28 ($p < .001$, 95% CI −.37, −.17). Both time required for an intervention and lack of referral resources remained serious concerns (see Figure 2).

Changes in SBIRT utilization at 3 months: Two hundred and twenty-seven providers (72%) reported that they conducted at least one intervention as part of the study. Providers were 30% more likely to use SBIRT than they had been at baseline. The effect of training on utilization was rated 7.8 for the workshop and 7.2 for the web on a scale of 1-10.

Predictors of utilization at 3 months: We used linear regression to identify predictors of increased SBIRT utilization, entering gender, profession, years in practice, and race and ethnicity, controlling for pre-test scores (see Figure 3). As years in practice increased, likelihood of SBIRT utilization increased (beta .015, $p < .001$, 95% CI .008, .021 adjusted R^2 .309). Demographics and type of profession (i.e., MD vs. RN vs. EMT) were not significant predictors of utilization.

Pre-Post Comparisons at 12 Months

Paired samples *t*-tests demonstrated sustained improvement over baseline in all domains except barriers (see Table 1). Enrollees who were followed were not significantly different in demographics or baseline composite scores from those lost to follow-up, but residents were less likely to be followed because many completed their training and moved away during the follow-up year.

Skills and responsibility at 12 months: Confidence in ability to perform SBIRT remained at 8% over baseline, but there was a 2% drop-off from the score at 3 months. Perception of responsibility to provide SBIRT held at 5% over baseline, but again dropped 2% from the 3 month score.

Barriers at 12 months: At post-test, barriers were not significantly different than at 3 months. Providers indicated continued belief that SBIRT would make a difference (3.74, $p < .001$, 95%CI −.26, −.01), a 3% increase over baseline but a 5% decline from the 3 month score.

SBIRT utilization at 12 months: Providers were 11% more likely to use SBIRT than at baseline, but there was a drop-off of 15% from the 3 month score.

Provider Comments

Successful experiences

(3 months post-training)

- I am shocked–patients are willing, and concerned about their ETOH problems. Because of my intervention with them I have had a very different rapport with my patients. We worked together. Again, I am amazed by the outcome.
- It takes a significant time commitment but it is important and worthwhile.

(12 months post-training)

- Patients seen much more responsive when using SBIRT. I found it surprisingly rewarding and patients were very receptive.
- So far, more patients than not have agreed to making some changes in their behavior.
- Often surprised how willing people are to agree to change and sign a contract to that effect.
- Patients are mostly very receptive to non-judgmental intervention.
- Patients seem responsive to counseling, especially if you show interest in the patient. Several patients have returned and mentioned that the interview was helpful.

TABLE 1. Changes in Provider Beliefs and Practices from Baseline to One Year Post Exposure to a Screening, Brief Intervention and Referral to Treatment Curriculum (SBIRT)*

Characteristic	Baseline	3 months	12 months
Confidence in ability to perform the elements of SBIRT	3.75	4.15 pre-post difference=0.40 p<.001, 95%CI -.50, -.32	4.06 pre-post difference=0.31 p<.002, 95%CI -.41, -.21
Responsibility to provide SBIRT	3.74	4.01 pre-post difference=0.25 p<.001, 95%CI -.33, -.17	3.91 pre-post difference=0.18 p<.04, 95%CI -.27, -.10
Barriers to Utilization of SBIRT	2.73	2.64 pre-post difference=0.09 p<.004, 95%CI -.03, -.15	2.65 pre-post difference=0.05 p=NS; 95%CI -.02, 13
Utilization of SBIRT	2.99	3.89 pre-post difference=0.90 p<.001, 95%CI -.98, -.83	3.32 pre-post difference=0.37 p<.001, 95%CI -.44, -.30

* values represent composite domain mean scores, with a scale range 1(least) to 5 (most)

FIGURE 2. Utilization and Perception of Barriers Over 12 Months

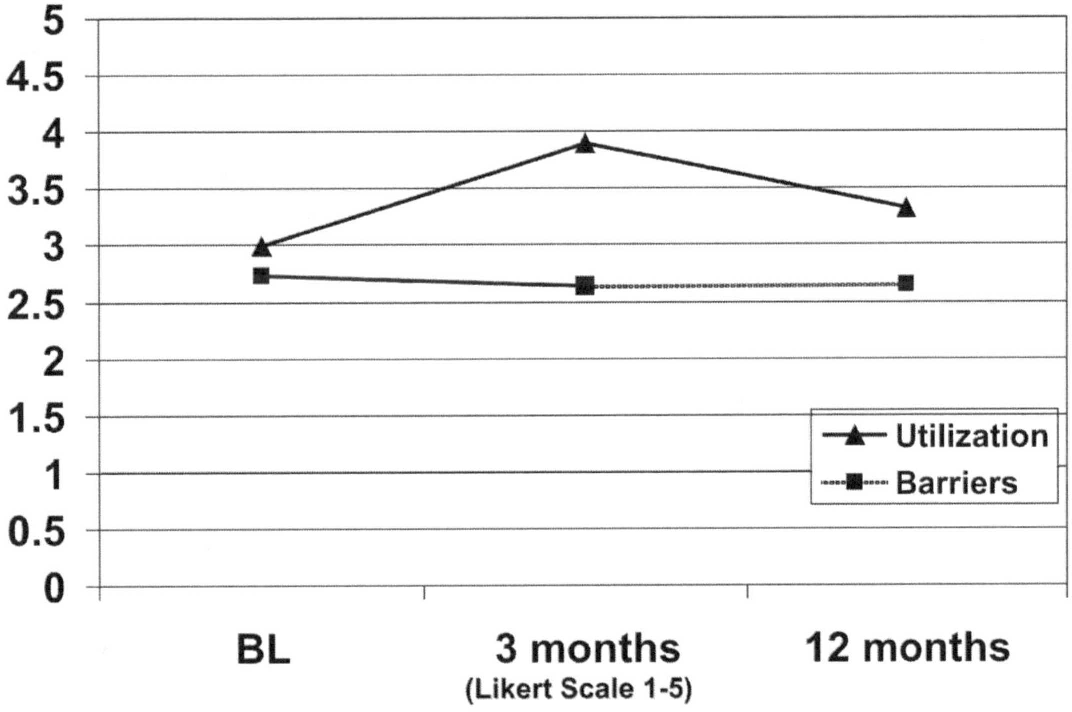

Barriers

- There is too much pressure from both attending MDs and Nurse Management to "move" and keep the patient "thru put" flowing for any of the nursing staff to perform an effective job in the alcohol screening. If we did do it correctly there would be criticism for not keeping up with the other patient acuity and overloading issues.
- I have had patients who are ready to change and sober and I cannot find a detox bed and at time of discharge from ER I send them with all the phone numbers and maybe a prescription for Ativan (if the MD will give one) and I feel as if I have failed them. It is like losing the one teachable moment.

Differences Among Sites

Among the 14 sites, three had pre-existing project ASSERT-type programs in which there were peer educators or trained extenders available in the ED to assist with referrals. At baseline, providers at these sites reported significantly higher means for ability (3.13 vs. 2.97, a difference of 0.16, $p < .05$, 95%CI .01, .31) and utilization (3.90 vs. 3.70, a difference of 0.20, $p < .05$, 95%CI .01, .39). While there were no differences in ability or utilization identified at follow-up, providers at the ASSERT sites were more likely to refer at 3 months (mean score 3.78 vs. 3.26, a difference of 0.52, $p < .001$, 95%CI −.78, −.26).

Comparison with Score Reported from the D'Onofrio et al. Controlled Trial, 2002

Mean composite scores were converted for comparability from a Likert scale of 1 to 5 to the 100 point scale reported in the previous study.[18] Baseline scores were somewhat higher in the present study, but improvements were comparable, and there was no significant difference in the percentages of pre-post improvement achieved in the two studies (Table 2).

DISCUSSION

ED providers at 14 academic sites across the country reported positive changes in their beliefs and clinical practices in response to exposure to a standardized SBIRT curriculum at 3 and 12 months. These findings involving 402 providers were very similar to previous findings by D'Onofrio et al. at one site. As reported

FIGURE 3. Likelihood of SBIRT Utilization Change with Years in Practice

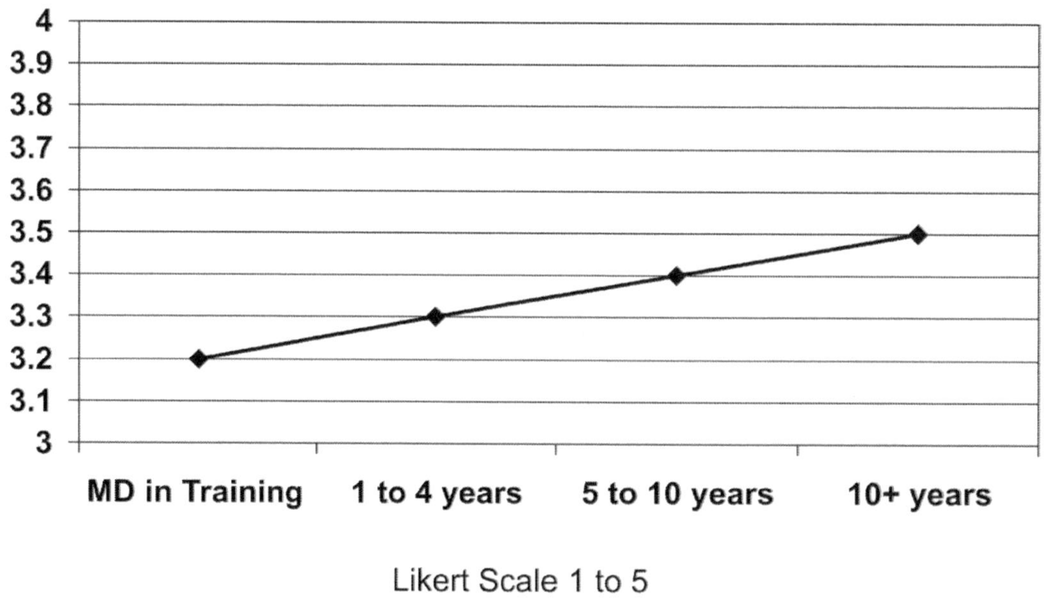

TABLE 2. Composite Mean Scores at Baseline and at 1 Year Follow-Up* Comparison with Controlled Trial, 2002[17]

	D'Onofrio et al. Intervention Site n = 17 (100% f/u rate)	% change in means pre/post	NASD ED SBIRT Collaborative n = 401 (72% f/u rate)	% change in means pre/post
Confidence	66.6 / 74.7	12	75.0 / 81.2	8
Responsibility	72.6 / 72.3	<1	74.8 / 78.2	5
Utilization	48.4 / 54.8	17	59.8 / 66.4	19

*scores scaled to 0-100
f/u=follow-up
NASD=National Alcohol Screening Day
ED=emergency Department
SBIRT=Screening, Brief Intervention and Referral to Treatment

in the survey results, these providers responded positively to SBIRT training, but recognized a need for institutional support and continued supervised clinical practice of SBIRT, and found that time constraints, reimbursement problems and lack of referral resources require major system changes. These barriers may explain why we observed only modest impact of the curriculum with attenuation evident at 12 months.

Nevertheless, there are many reasons for optimism. Thirty years ago internists did not recognize the importance of lipid screening and addressing diet and exercise behaviors. Today screening and recommendations for lifestyle behavior change are a standard of care. Emergency nursing and physician's professional organizations have supported National Alcohol Screening Day since 2000, and have endorsed policies to promote ED SBIRT. When this study was first announced in April 2003, Dr. Ting Kai Li, NIAAA Director, asserted that "Hospital EDs offer a unique opportunity not available elsewhere for alcohol abuse screening, brief counseling, and referral." Charles Curie, speaking for the Substance Abuse and Mental Health Administration (SAMHSA), added that "These efforts can reorient many people away from behaviors that, unchecked, can lead to addiction. For example, screening and referral to appropriate services for people who were driving while intoxicated could prevent repeat traumas and save countless lives." [33]

In this study, recognized ED leaders championed SBIRT nationally and in their own institutions. Also encouraging is the fact that ED providers who reported limited exposure to SBIRT in their ED training learned to go beyond the "found down" and "alcohol on breath" screening test to adopt a more standardized approach. The millions of ED patients with high risk and dependent drinking and those patients with frequent visits contribute to the high morbidity, mortality and costs and will continue to have a significant impact on the already stressed ED. Practical strategies to maximize efficient, effective approaches and to enhance patient and staff satisfaction were welcomed by providers, and this before and after study found that a relatively brief educational intervention was associated with small changes in confidence, responsibility and use of SBIRT by ED providers. It seems that more work is warranted to achieve greater changes in practices.

This evaluation of the impact of a standardized curriculum for providers was the companion piece to a trial of SBIRT among ED patients at these 14 sites. In this study, 2,051 ED patients (26% of those screened) exceeded the low-risk limits set by NIAAA; 1,132 consented and were enrolled (581 control, 551 intervention). At three month follow-up, patients receiving brief intervention by providers trained in the standardized curriculum reported significantly lower numbers of drinks per week (3.25) than controls, and were twice as likely as controls to be drinking under the NIAAA low-risk limit. This study demonstrated that an intervention by ED providers has some potential to reduce the alcohol consumption of ED patients and make an impact on alcohol-related morbidity, mortality and cost.[34]

Overall the educational effort was well received, and the learning curve was rapid. The curriculum offered an opportunity for ED residents to practice the Accreditation Council for Graduate Medical Education general core competencies for communication with patients, which state that ED professionals are expected to communicate effectively, demonstrate caring and respectful behaviors when interacting with patients and their families, counsel and educate patients and their families, and use effective listening skills.[35,36]

The concept of screening for alcohol use disorders or high risk drinking was easily accepted by ED practitioners, but universal screening takes time, and many drinkers are missed by targeted screening based on risk categories. NIAAA now recommends a single question that might be easily asked at triage: "How many times in the last month have you had 4 or more drinks on one occasion (for a female, or 5 or more for a male)?"

The intervention algorithm also contained many familiar elements taught as part of the medical interview. Patients were given feedback on the results of testing, the readiness ruler resembled pain scales commonly used in the ED, and patients received advice on how to avoid health consequences. The impact of the BNI on behavioral change is based on the fact that "the way clients are spoken to about changing addictive behavior affects their willingness to talk freely about why and how they might change."[37] Although professional feedback and advice and the teachable moment of an ED visit/personal crisis are powerful external motivators, they are not sufficient. Provider skills are necessary to facilitate and enhance internal motivation to change. Change is more likely, if patients can be assisted to name the problem and solution for themselves and come up with a workable/ efficacious plan that specifies concrete steps for addressing high risk and dependent drinking. In a number of cases referral will be needed, and ED providers will be more likely to refer if physician extenders, either peer counselors or social workers) are available to take the time that is required to ensure a successful placement for substance abuse.[38]

Furthermore, evidence has accumulated that patients exposed to SBIRT benefit from a booster session.[14] This study did not include any reinforcement after the formal training was concluded, and we should not be surprised by the drop-off in utilization at 12 months in the absence of a booster.

LIMITATIONS

Time available for the education program and intervention practice was limited by real-life conditions; SBIRT was one of many issues competing for the attention of residents. Changes observed in means were small, but still significant in a real-world setting. Because this study was intended as translational research, there was variation in practice from site to site, but training effects were still consistent across sites. Some residents were unavoidably lost to follow-up as they moved to take up new positions, but the follow-up rate was substantial at both three and 12 months, and those lost to follow-up were not different at baseline in prior training, demographics, confidence in ability or utilization of SBIRT. We would have liked to be able to evaluate the impact of independent study using the website, but our counter system did not allow us to link website users to study numbers. Some participants used the website in lieu of the workshop, while others used it as a booster, but we had no way to distinguish between these different modes. And of course, in a pre-post design without a control group, differences in outcomes may be confounded by secular trends or social desirability bias.

CONCLUSIONS

Exposure to an interactive screening, brief intervention and referral to treatment curriculum may increase competency and responsibility, decrease perceived barriers, and increase the likelihood of utilizing SBIRT. Training effects observed at three months persisted but were not sustained at the same level at 12 months. Resources such as computerized screening and the addition of ancillary support personnel to the ED team might increase the likelihood of SBIRT utilization. A booster workshop at six months might assist in sustaining changes in utilization.

REFERENCES

1. Harwood HJ. Updating estimates of economic costs of alcohol abuse in the United States: estimates, update methods, and data. Bethesda, MD. National Institute of Alcohol Abuse and Alcoholism, 2000.

2. Grant BF, Dawson DA, Stinson FS, Chou SP, Dufour MC, Pickering RP. The 12-month prevalence and trend in DSM-IV alcohol abuse and dependence, 1991-1992 and 2001-2002. Drug Alcohol Depend. 2004; 74:223-234.

3. Center for Disease Control. Alcohol-attributable deaths and years of potential life lost–United States 2001, MMWR Morb Mort Wkly Rep. 2004; 53; 866-870.

4. Brewer RD, Swahn MH. Binge drinking and violence. JAMA 2005; 294: 616-617.

5. McDonald AJ III, Wang N, Camargo CA Jr. US emergency department visits for alcohol-related diseases and injuries between 1992 and 2000. Arch Intern Med 2004; 164: 531-537.

6. Cherpitel CJ. Drinking patterns and problems: a comparison of primary care with the emergency room. Subst Abus. 1999; 20:85-95.

7. Bernstein E, Tracey A, Bernstein J, Williams C. Emergency Department detection and referral rates for patients with problem drinking. Subst Abuse 1996;17: 69-76.

8. Lowenstein SR, et al. Behavioral risk factors in Emergency Department Patients: A multi-site survey. Acad Emerg Med 1998; 5:781-787.

9. Cherpitel CJ. Screening for alcohol problems in the emergency department. Ann Emerg Med 1995; 26:158-166.

10. Davidson P, Koziol-McLain J, Harrison L, Timken D, Lowenstein S. Intoxicated ED patients: A five year follow-up of morbidity and mortality. Ann Emerg Med 1997; 30:593-597.

11. McCaig L, Burt CW. National Hospital Ambulatory Medical Care Survey. 2001emergency department summary. Advance data from vital and health statistics, no. 335. Hyattsville, MD: National Center for Health Statistics, 2003.

12. Results from the 2003 National Survey on Drug Use and Health: National Findings. Office of Applied Studies, Substance Abuse and Mental Health Services Administration. Available at: www.oas.samhsa.gov/nhsda/2k3nsduh/2k3Results.htm [accessed 10/9/05].

13. Whitlock EPM, Polen MRM, Green CAP, Orleans TP, Klein JM. Behavioral counseling interventions in primary care to reduce risky/harmful alcohol use by adults: a summary of the evidence for the U.S. Preventive Service Task Force. Ann Intern Med. 2004; 140:557-568.

14. Mello MJ, Nirenberg TD, Longabaugh R, Woolard R, Minugh A, Becker B et al. Emergency department brief motivational interventions for alcohol with motor vehicle crash patients. Ann Emerg Med. 2005; 45: 620-625.

15. Longabaugh R. Woolard RE, Nirenbereg TD, Evaluating the effects of a brief motivational intervention for injured drinkers in the emergency department. J Stud Alcohol. 2001; 62:806-816.

16. D'Onofrio GD, Degutis LC. Preventive care in the emergency department: screening and brief intervention for alcohol problems in the emergency department: a systematic review. Acad Emerg Med. 2002; 9: 627-638.

17. D'Onofrio G, Degutis LC, Fiellin DA, Pantalon MV, Busch SH, Chawarski MC, O'Connor PG. Emergency practitioner-performed brief interventions for harmful and hazardous drinkers in the emergency department. Acad Emerg Med 2002; 12 suppl 1: 59-60.

18. D'Onofrio G, Nadel ED, Degutis LC, Sullivan LM, Casper K, Bernstein E, Samet J. Improving emergency medicine residents' approach to patients with alcohol problems: A controlled educational trial. Ann Emerg Med. 2002; 40:50-62.

19. D'Onofrio GD, Pantalon MV, Degutis LC, Feillin DA, O'Connor PG. Development and implementation of an emergency department practitioner-performed brief intervention for hazardous and harmful drinkers in the emergency department. Acad Emerg Med. 2005; 12:211-218.

20. Davis DA, Thompson MA, Oxman ED, et al. Changing physician performance: A systematic review of the effect of medical education strategies. JAMA. 1995; 274:700-705.

21. Saitz R, Sullivan LM, Samet JH. Training community-based clinicians in screening and brief intervention for substance abuse problems: Translating evidence into practice. Substance Abuse. 2000;21:21-31.

22. The Physician Guide to Helping Patients with Alcohol Problems. Rockville, MD: National Institute of Alcohol Abuse and Alcoholism (NIAAA); U.S. Government Printing Office. 2004. (NIH Publication no. 4-3769)

23. Chafetz ME, et al. Establishing treatment relations with alcoholics. J Nerv Ment Dis 1962;134: 395-409.

24. Miller WR (ed.). Enhancing motivation for change in substance abuse, Treatment Improvement Protocol Series #35. US DHHS: Rockville, MD, 1999.

25. Miller WR, Rollnick S. Motivational Interviewing: Preparing People to Change Addictive Behaviors. New York: Guilford, 2002.

26. Prochaska JO, DiClemente C. Stages of change in the modification of problem behavior, in M. Hersen, R. Eisler and P. Miller, eds. Progress in behavior modification. Newbury Park, CA, Sage, 1992.

27. World Health Organization Brief Intervention Study Group. A cross national trial of brief interventions with heavy drinkers. Am J Pub Health 1996; 86: 948-955.

28. Bernstein E, Bernstein J, Levenson S. Project ASSERT: An ED-based intervention to increase access to primary care, preventive services, and the substance abuse treatment system. Ann Emerg Med. 1997; 30: 181-189.

29. D'Onofrio G, Bernstein E, Bernstein J. The Emergency Physician and the problem drinker. Boston: Marino Productions, 1998.

30. Amrhein PC, Miller WR, Yahne CE, Palmer M, Fulcher L. Client commitment language during motivational interviewing predicts drug use outcomes. J Consult Clin Psychol. 2003; 71:862-878.

31. Hettema J, Steele J, Miller WP. A meta-analysis of research on motivational interviewing treatment effectiveness. Ann Rev Clin Psych. 2005; 1:91-111.

32. SAMHSA. Substance Abuse Facility Locator. Available at: http://dasis3.samhsa.gov/ Accessibility verified August 17, 2005.

33. (NIH News Alcohol Agencies Announce Academic Emergency Medicine Department Collaboration. http://www.niaaa.nih.gov/press/2004/NASD04-04.htm)

34. Academic ED SBIRT Collaborative. The impact of screening, brief intervention and referral to treatment of emergency department patients' alcohol use. Ann Emerg Med. 2007 Sep 15; [Epub ahead of print].

35. ACGME Outcome Project. Accreditation Council for Graduate Medical Education. Available at http://www.acgme.org Accessibility verified August 17, 2005.

36. Hobgood CD, Riviello RJ, Jouriles N, Hamilton G. Assessment of communication and interpersonal skills competencies. Acad Emerg Med. 2002; 9: 1257-1269.

37. Rollnick S. Comments on Dunn et al.'s "The use of brief interventions adapted from motivational interviewing across behavioral domains: a systematic review." Enthusiasm, quick fixes and premature controlled trials. Addiction 2001; 96:1769-1770.

38. Bernstein E, Bernstein J. Commentary– SBIRT: Qualified trained assistants are necessary but not sufficient. Acad Emerg Med 2005; 12: 786-787.

doi:10.1300/J465v28n04_01

Brief Alcohol Interventions and Multiple Risk Factors in Primary Care

Jennifer S. Funderburk, PhD
Stephen A. Maisto, PhD
Dawn E. Sugarman, MS

SUMMARY. Early identification and intervention of harmful/hazardous drinking in primary care are U.S. healthcare priorities. Traditionally, research has focused on designing interventions for patients in primary care who report hazardous/harmful alcohol use, even though it is likely for a patient to be at risk for multiple problems. This article has three major goals: (1) to present data highlighting the prevalence and co-variation of other risk factors with hazardous/harmful drinking, including data from a small descriptive study; (2) to review the literature on brief alcohol interventions designed to address multiple risk factors; and (3) to provide recommendations for future research. Despite data indicating primary care patients present with multiple risk factors, only a limited number of studies in the literature have investigated brief interventions addressing alcohol use and other risk factors. It is important for future research to expand brief alcohol interventions to include other risk factors as well. doi:10.1300/J465v28n04_02 *[Article copies available for a fee from The Haworth Document Delivery Service: 1-800-HAWORTH. E-mail address: <docdelivery@haworthpress.com> Website: <http://www.HaworthPress.com> © 2007 by The Haworth Press, Inc. All rights reserved.]*

KEYWORDS. Alcohol, primary care, interventions, multiple risk, secondary prevention

A majority of adults are seen in primary care clinics every year (1). Thus, primary care is often characterized as the entry point to the U.S. health care system (2) and therefore provides an excellent opportunity for early intervention. Accordingly, primary care providers regularly screen for risk factors strongly linked with physical disease, which can be changed through behavioral modification and/or medication to significantly improve public health (2). For example, the primary care clinics within the U.S. Department of Veterans Affairs Health Care system regularly screen for several medical and mental health risk factors associated with hy-

Jennifer S. Funderburk, Stephen A. Maisto, and Dawn E. Sugarman are affiliated with the Center for Integrated Healthcare, Syracuse Veteran's Affairs Medical Center, and the Department of Psychology, Syracuse University, Syracuse, NY.

Jennifer S. Funderburk is also affiliated with the Department of Psychiatry, University of Rochester, Rochester, NY.

Address correspondence to: Jennifer S. Funderburk, Center for Integrated Healthcare, 800 Irving Avenue (116C), Syracuse, NY 13210 (E-mail: Jennifer.Funderburk@med.va.gov).

[Haworth co-indexing entry note]: "Brief Alcohol Interventions and Multiple Risk Factors in Primary Care." Funderburk, Jennifer S., Stephen A. Maisto, and Dawn E. Sugarman. Co-published simultaneously in *Substance Abuse* (The Haworth Medical Press, an imprint of The Haworth Press, Inc.) Vol. 28, No. 4, 2007, pp. 93-105; and: *Alcohol/Drug Screening and Brief Intervention: Advances in Evidence-Based Practice* (ed: Richard Saitz, and Marc Galanter) The Haworth Medical Press, an imprint of The Haworth Press, Inc., 2007, pp. 93-105. Single or multiple copies of this article are available for a fee from The Haworth Document Delivery Service [1-800-HAWORTH, 9:00 a.m. - 5:00 p.m. (EST). E-mail address: docdelivery@haworthpress.com].

Available online at http://suba.haworthpress.com

doi:10.1300/J465v28n04_02

pertension, heart disease, diabetes, and psychiatric disorders, like depression and alcohol abuse or dependence.

Due to the serious health risks posed by heavy alcohol use and the major consequences of alcohol-related problems for the United States economy (3), the U.S. Preventive Services Task Force recommended that primary care providers regularly screen for high risk drinking in their practices (4). Identifying and providing intervention in the primary care setting to patients who are hazardous and harmful drinkers is a current health care priority (2).

Hazardous and harmful drinkers include individuals who do not meet criteria for alcohol dependence, but whose alcohol use poses an increased risk for alcohol-related problems and/or whose drinking is associated with negative consequences. Research has shown that early intervention for hazardous or harmful drinking is efficacious when using brief alcohol interventions (5). These interventions are based on the belief that hazardous/harmful drinkers have the skills necessary to moderate their drinking. Therefore, the brief alcohol intervention is aimed at increasing the individual's motivation for or readiness to change his/her alcohol use (5, 6). Several reviews have found that brief alcohol interventions are efficacious in substantially reducing alcohol consumption when compared to no treatment or "standard care" control groups, and these effects are maintained for longer than a year (see 7-8 for reviews). For those individuals found to be alcohol dependent, current clinical guidelines recommend more intensive alcohol-related treatment, however brief intervention techniques could be used to help motivate an individual to engage in treatment (9).

With the advent of integrated healthcare models, the conceptual framework for the implementation of alcohol and other types of behavioral brief interventions is now available. Integrated healthcare models describe how behavioral health services can be integrated into the primary care environment. The overarching goal of these models is to help primary care providers treat the "whole" person by creating an environment consistent with the biopsychosocial approach (10), thereby eliminating many of the patient, provider, and system barriers that may prevent effective implementation of behavioral health services in traditional medical settings. These models describe how to establish collaborative, multidisciplinary teams focused on increasing the identification and detection of behavioral/psychological symptoms, like hazardous/harmful drinking, in the primary care setting (11). In fact, researchers have found that there is a higher level of treatment engagement in mental health services when an integrated healthcare model is used as compared to a model using enhanced referrals to specialty mental health care (12).

There are several models of integrated healthcare, and each model differs in its conceptualization of how to arrive at integration within the primary care system (10, 13-15). Although the models differ in their description of integration, a majority of them ultimately require the behavioral health provider to implement interventions that work in the context of primary care. Therefore, the format of interventions derived from these models may vary from interventions typically delivered in specialty mental health clinics. For instance, primary care interventions can be more team-based because the entire primary care team is on site and is actively involved in the patient's treatment. Additionally, interventions need to be brief (i.e., occur in 1-3 sessions, less than 30-minute meetings) to match the fast-paced nature of primary care as providers try to maintain a high level of accessibility to care for their patients, which is a vital component of primary care settings (16).

Another unique feature of primary care settings, in comparison to specialty mental health clinics, is how the primary care environment draws individuals who often have co-occurring risk factors and/or problems (2). These multiple co-morbidities further complicate the types of evidence-based interventions needed by behavioral health providers working in an integrated setting. Currently, efficacious brief alcohol interventions have been designed to reduce alcohol consumption and have typically not focused on any other types of risk factors that may often co-occur with hazardous/harmful alcohol use. Instead, research and program development have focused on understanding and constructing interventions for a single health risk factor, even though it is likely that an individual will report experiencing multiple risk factors (17). For instance, one study by Oslin and colleagues (18) examined a telephone disease management program for veterans exhibiting symptoms of depressive disorder and/or hazardous/harmful alcohol use. For those 11% of participants reporting co-morbid symptomatology, the research staff administered the two brief interventions designed for each disorder simultaneously while maintaining independent models of treatment. Therefore, research and interventions designed for individuals who present with co-morbidities or risk factors in primary care have been relatively neglected.

A major aim of this article is to review the prevalence and co-variation of multiple risk factors with harmful/hazardous alcohol use within primary care. Then, because of the lack of prevalence data examining harmful/hazardous alcohol use with other medical risk factors, like high blood pressure, we will present the findings of a descriptive study conducted to identify the prevalence and co-variation of multiple risk factors regularly assessed in a group of Department of Veterans Affairs (DVA) primary care clinics. After highlighting the need for brief interventions that focus on alcohol and other significant risk factors assessed in primary care, we review interventions in the literature that have addressed multiple risk factors including alcohol. This is followed by a discussion of the implications of our findings and suggestions for future research.

WHAT DO WE KNOW ABOUT THE PREVALENCE AND CO-VARIATION OF HAZARDOUS/ HARMFUL ALCOHOL USE AND OTHER RISK FACTORS IN PRIMARY CARE?

The tendency for risk factors to cluster together in one individual is not surprising, given that there is a dynamic interrelationship among behavior, biological changes, and risk for disease. For example, an individual's blood pressure is dependent on multiple factors, including family history of cardiovascular disease, smoking habits, alcohol use, physical activity, sodium intake, potassium intake, and diet (19). Because specific factors such as family history that contribute to risk cannot be modified, providers often focus on reducing risk by encouraging patients to change behaviors (e.g., take medication, reduce weight). Recent research has examined the prevalence of multiple risk factors by investigating behavioral risk factors identified as the four leading contributors to mortality: smoking, poor diet, sedentary behavior, and alcohol misuse (20). Using the National Health Interview data, Coups and colleagues (21) found that 52% of a sample of 16,818 participants reported two or more of the four behavioral risk factors. Examining the prevalence of these behavioral risk factors with high risk drinking, Rosal et al. (22) found that 67% of individuals identified as hazardous drinkers reported at least one other risk factor. The top five clusters of risk factors with hazardous drinking were: sedentary lifestyle (16%, i.e., not regularly exercising this past year); smoking (13%); smoking and sedentary lifestyle (10%); sedentary lifestyle and poor diet (10%); and smoking, sedentary lifestyle, and poor diet (8%).

Both of these studies provide data highlighting the prevalence of multiple risk factors and support the need for evidence-based interventions to address more than one risk factor. However, these studies examined risk factors that are not consistently screened for in primary care facilities in the United States. In fact, Coups et al. (21) found that approximately 30% of the participants indicated that their primary care provider never asked them about any of the four major behavioral risk factors cited earlier (i.e., smoking, diet, sedentary behavior, and alcohol use). Therefore, the study described next was designed to complement the Coups et al. (21) and Rosal et al. (22) research by providing data on the prevalence and co-variation of multiple risk factors regularly assessed within a group of DVA primary care clinics.

EXAMPLE: PREVALENCE OF MULTIPLE RISK FACTORS IN VISN 2 (UPSTATE NEW YORK) PRIMARY CARE CLINICS

Primary care clinics within Upstate New York Veteran's Integrated Service Network (VISN 2) regularly assess for the following: alcohol use, psychiatric distress including depression, body mass, smoking status, blood pressure, and cholesterol. This information is entered into the veteran's DVA electronic medical record by a health care provider, usually a licensed practical nurse. The DVA database can be scanned for relevant information contained in the DVA electronic medical record system and used for research purposes after obtaining IRB approval.

Participants

The DVA database was scanned and identified 86,326 veterans with a primary care encounter in VISN 2 from January 1st, 2005 to June 30th, 2005. Because not all of the patients had information recorded about their performance on the various screening measures, 15,356 patients were identified as having scores on all of the identified screening measures and were included in the analyses. Table 1 describes the demographic characteristics of this sub-sample of veterans.

Measures

The Alcohol Use Disorder Identification Test-C (*AUDIT-C*; 23, 24). The AUDIT-C is a

TABLE 1. Demographic Information for 15,356 VA Primary Care Patients.

Variable	Mean (*SD*)
Age	63.6 (13.8)
	N (%)
Married	9491 (61.8)
Male	14804 (96.4)
White	9418 (61.3)
Current Smoker	4441 (28.9)
ICD Diagnoses	*N (%)*
Hyperlipidemia	6865 (44.7)
Hypertension	9419 (61.3)
Coronary Artery Disease	3171(20.6)
Diabetes	3197 (20.8)
Stroke	574 (3.7)
Arthritis	3184 (20.7)
Depression	808 (5.3)
PTSD	848 (5.5)

3-item questionnaire that veterans are asked to complete annually and additionally as indicated clinically to screen for risk of alcohol problems.

The General Health Questionnaire (*GHQ*; 25). Veterans are asked to complete the GHQ annually and additionally as indicated clinically to assess for general psychiatric distress, including anxiety and depression.

Body mass index (BMI). *BMI* is calculated by adjusting the veteran's weight as a function of height using the following formula: (weight in kilograms)/(height in meters) (2).

Cholesterol screening. Cholesterol is measured from collecting information on the LDL and HDL values to screen for hyperlipidemia.

Blood pressure screening. Systolic and diastolic blood pressure (SBP and DBP, respectively) are measured at each primary care visit.

Tobacco use. Every year veterans are asked whether they are current smokers, or whether they quit less than 1 year ago, quit greater than 1 year ago, or never smoked.

Procedure

Demographic information and patient scores on the screening measures were identified and recorded for each veteran. Because many veterans had several values for each screening measure, we used the score on the AUDIT-C screen as a reference point, as that screen was our primary interest. Therefore, all of the other data were collected within 90 days of the AUDIT-C score.

Analyses

Because the primary objective of this study was to describe the prevalence and co-variation of multiple risk factors in this DVA patient sample, descriptive statistics were used. The first step was to determine if a patient was at-risk based on a specific screening measure; classification of a patient's risk status (positive or not) on a screening measure followed DVA clinical practice guidelines (26). Table 2 outlines the guidelines used to categorize veterans' scores on the various screening measures. Because the medical and psychosocial interventions used to modify systolic blood pressure (SBP) and diastolic blood pressure (DBP) are similar, the two blood pressure measures were combined. In contrast, medical interventions differ depending on the specific lipid value (LDL or HDL) labeled as at-risk; therefore, those values were kept as separate screening measures. Recently, the guidelines for the

TABLE 2. The Categorization of the Screening Measures Based on the VA Guidelines

Screening Measure	Negative	Positive ("at-risk")
AUDIT-C	< 4	≥ 4
GHQ	< 4	≥ 4
BMI	$18.5 \geq \text{BMI} < 25$	$\text{BMI} \geq 25$ or $\text{BMI} < 18.5$
Blood Pressure	$\text{SBP} < 120$ and $\text{DBP} < 80$	$\text{SBP} \geq 120$ or $\text{DBP} \geq 80$
Smoking Status	Never or Former Smoker	Current Smoker
LDL value	< 130	≥ 130
HDL value	≥ 40	< 40

at-risk cholesterol values were changed to depend on the individual's 10 year risk of a cardiac event. To be conservative, we chose an LDL value that would be considered at-risk if the veteran had a moderate risk of cardiac events (i.e., 10 year risk of a cardiac event is 10%). We then calculated a summary score to reflect the number of positive screening measures scores for each veteran. Using frequency counts, we examined the number of screening measures veterans scored positive independently and then the prevalence of the different combination of screening measures.

Results

Table 3 shows the frequencies of veterans scoring positive on each individual screening measure. To help understand the prevalence of veterans having multiple risk factors, Table 4 shows the prevalence of veterans with zero to seven positive screens. A small percentage (2%) of the sample met all of the guidelines with no positive screens. However, a large percentage of the sample had two or more risk factors (84%), and more than half of the sample had three of more risk factors (53%). Moreover, it was common for patients with a positive AUDIT-C screen to also have multiple co-occuring risk factors. As shown in Table 5, approximately 96% of patients with a positive AUDIT-C screen also had at least one co-occurring risk factor, and 75% of AUDIT-C positive patients had two or more co-occuring risk factors.

To determine the most prevalent combinations of positive screens, we focused on the combinations of positive screens involving four screens or fewer, because they accounted for 93% of the sample. Then, the most prevalent combinations of positive screens (i.e., the top 25% of the combinations) were identified by using the 3rd quartile as the cut-off point. Table 6 shows the top ten combinations of these positive screens. The alcohol screen appears in three of the top ten combinations, indicating that 10% of the sample screened positive on the AUDIT-C combined with the BMI, BP, or HDL screens.

Summary

These DVA VISN 2 data are consistent with those of previous studies in showing the high frequency of primary care patients having multiple risk factors. In addition, this study highlights the co-variation of those individuals who screened positive for hazardous/harmful alcohol use with other screens regularly assessed in primary care, including body mass index, high

TABLE 3. Number and Percentage of Veterans Scoring Positive on Each Screening Measure

Screening Measure	*N*	Percent of total sample
BMI	12625	82.2
HDL value	6988	45.5
Blood Pressure	5804	37.8
AUDIT-C	5170	33.7
Smoking Status	4441	28.9
LDL value	4218	27.5
GHQ	1597	10.4

Note: N = 15,356

TABLE 4. The Frequency and Percent of Patients with a Specific Number of Positive Screens

Number of Positive Screens	*N*	Percent	Cumulative Percent
7	15	0.1	0.1
6	168	1.1	1.2
5	825	5.4	6.6
4	2488	16.2	22.8
3	4694	30.6	53.4
2	4751	30.9	84.3
1	2069	13.5	97.8
0	346	2.3	100.0

Note: The seven screening measures included were: BMI, HDL value, LDL value, blood pressure, AUDIT-C, smoking status, and GHQ. Total $N = 15{,}356$

TABLE 5. The Frequency and Percent of Patients Scoring Positive on the AUDIT-C with a Specific Number of Other Positive Screens

Number of Positive Screens with a Positive AUDIT-C	*N*	Percent	Cumulative Percent
6	0	0	0
5	137	2.6	2.6
4	558	10.8	13.4
3	1388	26.8	40.3
2	1768	34.2	74.5
1	1095	21.2	95.7
0	194	3.8	100.0

Note: The screening measures included were: BMI, HDL value, LDL value, blood pressure, smoking status, and GHQ. Total $N = 5{,}170$

TABLE 6. The Top Ten Most Prevalent Clusters of Positive Multiple Risk Factor Screens

Combinations of Screening Measures	Number of Unique Individuals	Percent of Total Sample ($N = 15{,}356$)
BMI & HDL	1620	10.55
BMI, HDL, & BP	944	6.15
BMI & BP	754	4.91
AUDIT-C & BMI	678	4.42
AUDIT-C, BMI, & BP	506	3.30
BMI, Smoking, & HDL	487	3.17
BMI & LDL	468	3.05
AUDIT-C, BMI, & HDL	416	2.71
BMI, LDL, & HDL	392	2.55
BMI, LDL, & BP	335	2.18

blood pressure, and high-density lipoprotein. Unlike the study of Rosal et al. (22), this study focused on risk factors regularly measured and monitored in primary care clinics (e.g., blood pressure, cholesterol). Like the behavioral risk factors in Rosal et al.'s (22) study, these biological risk factors are often addressed through behavioral changes and/or medication. For example, low-density lipoprotein, a form of cholesterol, can be decreased through the use of medication, diet changes, and/or exercise (27). High blood pressure is generally reduced through the use of medication, exercise, and/or diet changes (19). Whether the patient is prescribed a new medication or needs to change his/her behavior, these data highlight the need for brief interventions focused on changing more than one behavior for those patients identified at risk for multiple problems.

ARE THERE BRIEF ALCOHOL INTERVENTIONS DESIGNED TO ADDRESS OTHER RISK FACTORS?

A literature review was performed to examine the types of brief interventions designed for adults that address alcohol and other risk factors identified as common in primary care settings. Five studies were identified as multiple risk interventions including alcohol (28-32). Four of the studies were randomized controlled trials (28, 29, 31, 32), and one study used ad hoc non randomized comparison (30). This review focuses on describing the characteristics of these interventions.

Three of the intervention studies focused on cardiovascular risk, but contained an alcohol risk component (29, 30, 32). All three studies provided some feedback to participants (either individualized or general) about the risk associated with alcohol use and included discussion of behavior change. However, alcohol use was discussed in relation to cardiovascular risk, and participants were not screened for hazardous drinking. Thus, participants in these samples included abstainers and light drinkers as well as hazardous/harmful drinkers and/or those who are alcohol dependent. Overall, these three interventions focused on cardiovascular risk and found significant results for lowered cardiovascular risk (32), increased self-reported lifestyle changes (30), and decreased blood pressure, fasting lipids, and obesity parameters (weight, BMI, and waist circumference) (29) in the intervention group compared to the control group. Of note, the study by Emmen and colleagues (30) found that, although more intervention participants than control participants reported making lifestyle changes, only 51% of participants reporting lifestyle changes showed clinically significant behavior change. Furthermore, two of the studies did not report outcome results related to alcohol use (30, 32), and the third study found no group differences in alcohol consumption from baseline to follow-up (29).

The last two studies relating to multiple risk interventions including alcohol use were not specifically focused to a certain disease. One of the studies was designed to address three health behaviors that have been shown to be risks for a variety of illnesses: smoking, excessive alcohol use, and sedentary lifestyle (28) in participants aged 65 and over. Intervention participants received two preventative examinations in which their primary care physician reviewed lifestyle health behaviors with them (i.e., smoking, exercise, diet, alcohol use/abuse, emotional distress, injury prevention, sleep problems, medication use, functional status, and urinary incontinence). Although the proportion of smokers and problem drinkers declined overall at the two-year follow-up visit, results showed no effect of the intervention on improvement of any of the three risk behaviors (smoking, alcohol use, and sedentary lifestyle).

The last study investigated a web-based primary care intervention for multiple health risk behaviors in patients attending a student health center in New Zealand (31). The intervention group received personalized feedback on physical activity, fruit and vegetable intake, alcohol consumption, and smoking, and health authority recommendations were given for each of these behaviors. Results indicated that participants in the feedback group had significantly greater compliance with the recommendations for fruit and vegetable consumption and physical activity compared to a minimal contact group. In addition, there were no significant group differences in compliance with the alcohol use recommendations.

CONCLUSION

In summary, few studies have investigated brief interventions addressing alcohol use and other risk factors. Of those studies identified, the majority included alcohol as only a component of the intervention and did not target participants who were hazardous/harmful drinkers. Instead, the studies either targeted the intervention to those patients with a high level of cardiovascular risk or provided the intervention to a non-targeted sample of patients. Two studies did not report results specific to alcohol (30, 32), and the other three studies reported no significant alcohol use outcomes for the intervention group versus control or comparison groups (28, 29, 31).

The variability in the content of the interventions is considerable, with several interventions focused on providing non-individualized health education regarding the lifestyle factors associated with cardiovascular risk (29, 32) to other studies providing personalized feedback about the individual's behaviors, including alcohol use (28, 30, 31). Additionally, the formats of the interventions ranged from individual sessions with the primary care provider (28) to written or web-based feedback (30, 31) to a combination of lectures and classes (29). Lastly, these interventions ranged in number of sessions and duration. Examples of two of the briefest interventions were the study by Kypri and McAnally (31) that consisted of one session in which participants received personalized feedback and advice via the web, and the study by Emmen and colleagues (30) in which participants received written feedback plus brief physician advice. Examples of two of the longer interventions were the study by Cakir and Pinar (29) in which participants attended four psychoeducational classes and received individual counseling, and the study by Wood and colleagues (32) in which participants received personalized feedback and 1-6 follow-up visits.

WHAT ARE THE NEXT STEPS?

It is clear that multiple risk factors are prevalent in the primary care setting. This article presented data indicating that individuals identified as "at risk" (for alcohol problems) drinkers were likely to have other significant behavioral and medical risk factors. However, a review of the literature demonstrated that only a few studies have examined brief interventions for multiple risk factors that included alcohol. More importantly, these studies were not designed to act as an early intervention for patients identified in primary care as at-risk following positive screening results.

As behavioral health providers begin to work in integrated primary care settings, there is a greater likelihood that brief behavioral interventions can be implemented in primary care to address these behavioral and medical risk factors. In addition, brief behavioral interventions complement the regular screening process present within the primary care setting by offering preventative behavioral interventions to patients identified as at-risk. Preventative interventions may be helpful to providers treating patients who present with sub-threshold symptomatology, for which medication may not be recommended. For instance, patients exhibiting pre-hypertensive levels of blood pressure and/or hazardous/harmful drinking are often recommended to make behavioral changes, including: reduction of alcohol use, diet changes, and/or exercise (19).

It is important to note that it is unreasonable to expect providers to deliver unique interventions for each medical and behavioral risk factor identified in every patient, especially because many patients' exhibit clusters of risk factors as described earlier. Because behavioral health providers operate as members of the primary care team in integrated primary care settings, interventions need to be sensitive to the time constraints often present within the primary care setting. Therefore, a brief intervention that addresses more than one risk factor would fit more easily into the fast-paced nature of primary care and would better match the heterogeneous presentation of patients in the private sector. Primary care providers in the United States tend to work within 15-minute visits, and integrated healthcare models often describe behavioral health providers' limiting their encounters with patients to one-three 30-minute visits (15). Therefore, the intervention must be able to fit within those limitations of the primary care team. Currently, brief alcohol interventions for primary care range in time commitments from one, 5-10 minute session with 2 booster follow-up phone calls to a 45 minute session with 2 booster follow-up phone calls (33-39). These efficacious brief alcohol interventions clearly demonstrate that some brief interventions are a good match with the time limitations of primary care, but these interventions need to be expanded to address the common occurrence of patients with more than one risk factor.

One way to maintain the brief nature of these interventions while addressing multiple risk factors is to construct interventions that take advantage of the collaborative, team-based nature of primary care. This is dramatically different than individual sessions at a specialty mental health setting, where brief interventions can also be applied. Additionally, brief interventions can take advantage of the established relationships between the patient and the primary care team, which may also increase the impact of the intervention. Because primary care providers remain fairly consistent across time, patients have the opportunity to strengthen their relationships every time the patient returns for a visit. Therefore, brief interventions can take advantage of these established relationships by incorporating them into the intervention to not only reduce the time any one provider spends with the patient, but also increase the impact. For instance, a brief intervention may incorporate a joint 5-minute session, where the primary care provider and behavioral health provider work together explaining the relationships among the different risk factors the patient is reporting and the implications both medically and psychologically to the patient.

Addressing more than one risk factor at a time within a brief intervention also provides the opportunity to acknowledge the relationships among the risk factors. Many of the behavioral and biological factors screened for within a primary care setting, as signs of disease, are related to one another through underlying biological mechanisms unknown to most patients. For instance, high blood pressure is linked with aspects of diet, alcohol use, exercise, and smoking (19). Delivering interventions sequentially that address only one risk factor at a time ignores how these risk factors are interconnected. An intervention designed to address co-existing risk factors using a single integrated model may be more effective because it highlights how each risk factor affects the other (40). For hazardous/harmful alcohol use, covariation among medical and behavioral problems can easily be discussed when addressing other risk factors such as cholesterol level, blood pressure, diet, or depression.

Beyond the underlying biological connections between medical and biological risk factors commonly screened for within primary care, there is also a common thread related to the implication that a patient needs to change his/her behaviors to reduce the risk. Whether the intervention is focused on increasing the individual's medication compliance, reducing his/her alcohol use, or changing his/her diet, behavior interventions often focus on increasing an individual's readiness to change. Therefore, as brief alcohol interventions incorporate additional risk factors, the focus on readiness to change will most likely be a common theme when discussing the patient's risk factors.

Because brief interventions cannot be developed to address all of the potential combinations between hazardous/harmful alcohol use and the other risk factors, it may be prudent for researchers to use epidemiological/descriptive data to identify those clusters of risk factors most prevalent in the primary care population. This would result in brief alcohol interventions being expanded to include other risk factors based on actual population needs. For example, based on the data presented earlier, further examination of interventions addressing alcohol use and weight or alcohol use and blood pressure may be useful within the DVA primary care system.

However, the question of whether a brief intervention for multiple risk factors is as effective for improving alcohol and other health outcomes as providing the brief intervention targeting alcohol consumption alone has not been answered. The literature review conducted in this paper provides no evidence regarding this question. Other studies provide some hope for the success of multiple risk factor interventions in reducing multiple targeted risk factors. For instance, the Multiple Risk Factor Intervention Trial (41) demonstrated a decline in mean risk factor levels (i.e., smoking, blood pressure, and cholesterol) targeted in the intervention, even 1 year after study completion, as compared to the usual care group. Additionally, it may be the case that certain risk factors can be treated by use of a single intervention, and other risk factors need to be targeted by interventions independently. Therefore, further exploration on which risk factors, not only are prevalent in the population, but also may be addressed simultaneously is needed.

In sum, this article has highlighted several future directions for researchers in regard to program development. As integrated healthcare models become more popular in the primary care setting, further opportunities are created to provide early identification and intervention. Due to the increased likelihood of the co-occurrence of multiple risk factors with hazardous/harmful drinking, it is important for brief alcohol interventions implemented in the primary care setting to be expanded to address other risk factors as well.

REFERENCES

1. Hing EP, Cherry DK, Woodwell DA. National Ambulatory Medical Care Survey: 2004 Summary. Advance Data from Vital and Health Statistics. Vol. 374. Hyattsville, MD: National Center for Health Statistics, pp. 1-36, 2006.

2. Institute of Medicine. Alcohol problems: Broadening the base of treatment. Washington, DC: National Academy Press, 1990.

3. Schneider Institute for Health Policy. Substance abuse: The nation's number one health problem. In: Foundation RWJ, ed. Waltham, MA: Brandeis University, 2001.

4. U.S. Preventive Services Task Force. Screening and behavioral counseling interventions in primary care

to reduce alcohol misuse: Recommendation statement. Annals of Internal Medicine 2004; 140: 554-556.

5. Kavanagh DJ, Sitharthan T, Spilsbury G, Vignaedra S. Effectiveness of physician-based interventions with problem drinkers: A review. Behavior Therapy 1999; 30: 641-656.

6. Davidson R. Facilitating change in problem drinkers. In: Davidson R, Rollnick S, MacEwan I, eds. Counselling Problem Drinkers. New York, NY: Tavistock/Routledge, pp. 3-20, 1991.

7. Bertholet N, Daeppen JB, Wietlisbach V, Fleming M, Burnand B. Reduction of alcohol consumption by brief alcohol intervention in primary care: Systematic review and meta-analysis. Archives of Internal Medicine. 2005; 165: 986-995.

8. Whitlock EP, Polen MR, Green CA, Orleans T, Klein J. Behavioral counseling interventions in primary care to reduce risky/harmful alcohol use by adults: A summary of the evidence for the U.S. Preventive Services Task Force. Annals of Internal Medicine. 2004; 140: 557-568.

9. Moyer A, Finney JW. Brief interventions for alcohol problems: Factors that facilitate implementation. Alcohol Research & Health 2004; 28(1): 44-50.

10. Blount A. Integrated primary care: Organizing the evidence. Families, Systems & Health 2003; 21: 121-133.

11. O'Donohue WT, Byrd MR, Cummings NA, Henderson DA, eds. Behavioral Integrative Care: Treatments that Work in the Primary Care Setting. New York, NY: Brunner-Routledge, 2005.

12. Bartels SJ, Coakley EH, Zubritsky C, Ware JH, Miles KM, Areán PA, Chen H, Oslin D, Llorente MD, Costantino G, Quijano L, McIntyre JS, Linkins KW, Oxman TE, Maxwell J, Levkoff SE. Improving access to geriatric mental health services: A randomized trial comparing treatment engagement with integrated versus enhanced referral care for depression, anxiety, and at-risk alcohol use. American Journal of Psychiatry 2004; 161: 1455-1462.

13. Doherty WJ. The why's and levels of collaborative family health care. Family Systems Medicine 1995; 13: 275-281.

14. Dym B, Berman S. The primary health care team: Family physician and family therapist in joint practice. Family Systems Medicine 1986; 4: 9-21.

15. Strosahl K. Integrating behavioral health and primary care services: The primary mental health care model. In: Blount A, ed. Integrated Primary Care: The Future of Medical and Mental Health Collaboration. New York, NY: W.W. Norton & Co., pp. 139-166, 1998.

16. Robinson P. Adapting empirically supported treatments to the primary care setting: A template for success. In: O'Donohue WT, Byrd MR, Cummings NA, Henderson DA, eds. Behavioral Integrative Care: Treatments that Work on the Primary Care Setting. New York, NY: Brunner-Routledge, 2005.

17. Pronk NP, Peek CJ, Goldstein MG. Addressing multiple behavioral risk factors in primary care. A synthesis of current knowledge and stakeholder dialogue sessions. Am J Prev Med 2004; 27: 4-17.

18. Oslin DW, Sayers S, Ross J, Kane V, Have TT, Conigliaro J, Cornelius J. Disease management for depression and at-risk drinking via telephone in an older population of veterans. Psychosomatic Medicine 2003; 65: 931-937.

19. Whelton PK, He J, Appel LJ, Cutler JA, Havas S, Kotchen TA, Roccella EJ, Stout R, Vallbona C, Winston MC, Karimbakas J. Primary prevention of hypertension: Clinical and public health advisory from the national high blood pressure education program. JAMA 2002; 288: 1882-1888.

20. McGinnis JM, Foege WH. Actual causes of death in the United States. JAMA 1993; 270: 2207-2212.

21. Coups EJ, Gaba A, Orleans CT. Physician screening for multiple behavioral health risk factors. American Journal of Preventive Medicine 2004; 27: 34-41.

22. Rosal MC, Ockene JK, Hurley TG, Reiff S. Prevalence and co-occurrence of health risk behaviors among high-risk drinkers in a primary care population. Preventive Medicine: An International Journal Devoted to Practice and Theory 2000; 31: 140-147.

23. Saunders JB, Aasland OG, Babor TF, de la Fuente JR, Grant M. Development of the alcohol use disorders identification test (AUDIT): WHO collaborative project on early detection of persons with harmful alcohol consumption: II. Addiction 1993; 88: 791-804.

24. Dawson DA, Grant BF, Stinson FS, Zhou Y. Effectiveness of the derived alcohol use disorders identification test (AUDIT-C) in screening for alcohol use disorders and risk drinking in the US general population. Alcoholism: Clinical and Experimental Research 2005; 29: 844-854.

25. Goldberg DG. Manual of the general health questionnaire. Windsor: NFER Publishing, 1978.

26. Office of Quality and Performance. Clinical Practice Guidelines, 2006.

27. McKenney JM. Lipid management: Tools for getting to the goal. American Journal of Managed Care 2001; 7: S299-306.

28. Burton LC, Paglia MJ, German PS, Shapiro S, Damiano AM. The effect among older persons of general preventive visit on three health behaviors: Smoking, excessive alcohol drinking, and sedentary lifestyle. Preventive Medicine 1995; 24: 492-497.

29. Cakir H, Pinar R. Randomized controlled trial on lifestyle modification in hypertensive patients. Western Journal of Nursing Research 2006; 28: 190-209.

30. Emmen MJ, Peters E, Elving LD, Bredie SJH, Wollersheim H, Bleijenberg G, Schippers GM. A brief behavioral feedback intervention in hospital outpatients with a high cardiovascular risk. Patient Education and Counseling 2006; 60: 32-40.

31. Kypri K, McAnally HM. Randomized controlled trial of a web-based primary care intervention for multiple health risk behaviors. Preventive Medicine 2005; 41: 761-766.

32. Wood DA, Kinmonth AL, Davies GA, Yarwood J, Thompson SG, Pyke SDM, Kok Y, Cramb R, Le Guen C, Marteau TM, Durrington PN. Randomised controlled trial evaluating cardiovascular screening and intervention in general practice: Principal results of British family heart study. British Medical Journal 1994; 308: 313-320.

33. Fleming MF, Manwell LB, Barry KL, Adams W, Stauffacher EA. Brief physician advice for alcohol problems in older adults: A randomized community-based trial. Journal of Family Practice 1999; 48: 378-384.

34. Curry SJ, Ludman EJ, Grothaus LC, Donovan D, Kim E. A randomized trial of a brief primary-care based intervention for reducing at-risk drinking practices. Health Psychology 2003; 22: 156-165.

35. Fleming MF, Barry KL, Manwell LB, Johnson K, London. Brief physician advice for problem alcohol drinkers: A randomized controlled trial in community-based primary care practices. JAMA 1997; 277: 1039-1045.

36. WHO Brief Intervention Study Group. A cross-national trial of brief interventions with heavy drinkers. American Journal of Public Health 1996; 86: 948-955.

37. Burge SK, Amodei N, Elkin B, Catala S, Andrew S. An evaluation of two primary care interventions for alcohol abuse among Mexican-American patients. Addiction 1997; 92: 1705-1716.

38. Senft RA, Polen MR, Freeborn DK, Hollis JF. Brief intervention in a primary care setting for hazardous drinkers. American Journal of Preventive Medicine 1997; 13: 464-470.

39. Maisto SA, Conigliaro JC, McNeil M, Kraemer K, Conigliaro RL, Kelley ME. Effects of two types of brief interventions and readiness to change on alcohol use in hazardous drinkers. Journal of Studies on Alcohol 2001; 62: 605-614.

40. Weiss R, Najavits L. Overview of treatment modalities for dual diagnosis patients: Pharmacotherapy, psychotherapy, and 12-step programs. In: Kranzler H, Rounsaville B, eds. Dual Diagnosis and Treatment: Substance Abuse and Comorbid Medical and Psychiatric Disorders. New York: Marcel Dekker Inc., pp. 87-105, 1998.

41. Multiple Risk Factor Intervention Trial Research Group. Multiple risk factor intervention trial: Risk factor changes and mortality results. Journal of the American Medical Association 1982; 248: 1465-1477.

doi:10.1300/J465v28n04_02

Adolescents' Preferences for Substance Abuse Screening in Primary Care Practice

John R. Knight, MD
Sion K. Harris, PhD
Lon Sherritt, MPH
Shari Van Hook, MPH
Nohelani Lawrence, BS
Traci Brooks, MD
Peggy Carey, MD
Robert Kossack, MD
John Kulig, MD, MPH

John R. Knight, Sion K. Harris, Lon Sherritt, and Shari Van Hook are affiliated with the Department of Pediatrics, Harvard Medical School, and the Center for Adolescent Substance Abuse Research, Children's Hospital Boston, Boston, MA.

Nohelani Lawrence is affiliated with the Center for Adolescent Substance Abuse Research, Children's Hospital Boston, Boston, MA.

Traci Brooks is affiliated with the Department of Pediatrics, Harvard Medical School, Boston, MA and the Cambridge Health Alliance, Cambridge, MA.

Peggy Carey is affiliated with Milton Family Practice, Milton, VT and the University of Vermont College of Medicine, Burlington, VT.

Robert Kossack is affiliated with Fallon Clinic, Worcester, MA.

John Kulig is affiliated with the Department of Pediatrics, Tufts New England Medical Center Floating Hospital for Children, Boston, MA.

Address correspondence to: John R. Knight, MD, Director, Center for Adolescent Substance Abuse Research, Children's Hospital Boston, 300 Longwood Avenue, Boston, MA 02115 (E-mail: john.knight@childrens.harvard.edu) (Web: http://www.ceasar.org/).

The authors thank the physicians and staff of The New England Partnership for Substance Abuse Research for assistance with study implementation, including Kathleen Kelley, MBA; Jeanne McBride, RN, BSN, MM, Quality Improvement Project Manager, UMMHC Department of Family Medicine and Community Health; Irene Phelps, RN, BSN; Judy Shaw, RN, MPH, Executive Director, Vermont Child Health Improvement Program; Donald H. Taylor III, MIT; and Colleen Sheppard, RN, BSN, Division of General Pediatrics and Adolescent Medicine, Tufts-New England Medical Center.

This study was supported by grant # 45222 from The Robert Wood Johnson Foundation. Other support was provided by Grant K07 AA013280 from the National Institute on Alcohol Abuse and Alcoholism (JRK) and Grant #5T20MC000-11-06 (SVH, JRK) and grant #5T71MC00009-12-0 (SKH) from the Maternal and Child Health Bureau.

No author or immediate family member has a financial relationship or interest with any proprietary entity producing health care goods or services related to the content of this report. This paper does not include discussion of or reference to any commercial products or services, and it does not discuss an unapproved or investigative use of any commercial products/devices.

[Haworth co-indexing entry note]: "Adolescents' Preferences for Substance Abuse Screening in Primary Care Practice." Knight, John R. et al. Co-published simultaneously in *Substance Abuse* (The Haworth Medical Press, an imprint of The Haworth Press, Inc.) Vol. 28, No. 4, 2007, pp. 107-117; and: *Alcohol/Drug Screening and Brief Intervention: Advances in Evidence-Based Practice* (ed: Richard Saitz, and Marc Galanter) The Haworth Medical Press, an imprint of The Haworth Press, Inc., 2007, pp. 107-117. Single or multiple copies of this article are available for a fee from The Haworth Document Delivery Service [1-800-HAWORTH, 9:00 a.m. - 5:00 p.m. (EST). E-mail address: docdelivery@haworthpress.com].

Available online at http://suba.haworthpress.com

doi:10.1300/J465v28n04_03

SUMMARY. *Objective:* To assess adolescents' preferences for substance abuse screening in primary medical care settings.

Design/Methods: Twelve- to 18-year-old patients (N = 2133) arriving for routine care at a network of primary care sites completed an interview that included demographic items, the CRAFFT screen, and a questionnaire assessing preferences for screening method (paper questionnaire, computer, oral interview by nurse or doctor). A subgroup (n = 222) completed the CRAFFT directly on the computer.

Results: Across the entire sample, paper was the screening administration method most preferred (mean rank (MR) = 2.92, 95%CI 2.87-2.96) vs. computer (MR = 2.38, 2.33-2.43), nurse (MR = 2.43, 2.39-2.47), and doctor (MR = 2.30, 2.25-2.35). Among the participants who received the screening on the computer, however, computer (MR = 3.08, 95%CI 2.42-2.52) was statistically tied with paper (MR = 2.88, 2.75-3.02) and both were ranked significantly higher than nurse (MR = 2.06, 1.94-2.17) and doctor (MR = 1.98, 1.82-2.14). The findings were similar for participants' reports of being "very likely" to be honest when answering substance abuse screening questions.

Conclusions: Adolescents should ideally be screened for substance abuse using paper or computer questionnaires. doi:10.1300/J465v28n04_03

KEYWORDS. Substance-related disorders, alcoholism, adolescence, screening, questionnaire, drug abuse detection

INTRODUCTION

Substance misuse by adolescents continues to be one of the nation's leading public health problems. According to the University of Michigan's annual Monitoring the Future Study, 80% of students have begun to drink and 50% have used an illicit drug by senior year in high school (1). Alcohol use is linked to accidents, homicides, and suicides, which are the leading causes of death among teenagers in the United States (2). Early age of onset of drinking is associated with a greatly increased risk of developing alcohol dependence later in life (3). In addition, alcohol and drug use are associated with a wide variety of other health risks and problems (4-7), making settings where adolescents receive routine health care ideal for implementation of substance abuse screening and early intervention programs (8-10).

National practice guidelines recommend that all adolescent patients be screened for substance use during the annual well care visit (9,11), and it may be even more important to screen during sick visits and urgent care encounters. A variety of screening tests have been validated in adolescent populations, including the CRAFFT questions (12), the Problem Oriented Screening Instrument for Teenagers (POSIT) (13), and the Alcohol Use Disorders Identification Test (AUDIT) (14). Among these, the CRAFFT was specifically developed to be practical for busy primary care practices; it is brief and easy to score. Prior studies have shown that the CRAFFT is developmentally appropriate for adolescents, capable of identifying need for substance abuse treatment, and sufficiently sensitive and specific for identifying substance-related problems and disorders (15,16).

CRAFFT is a conjoint screen (i.e., screens for alcohol and drugs simultaneously) comprised of six questions. "Have you ever ridden in a CAR driven by someone (including yourself) who was 'high' or had been using alcohol or drugs? Do you ever use alcohol or drugs to RELAX, feel better about yourself, or fit in? Do you ever use alcohol or drugs while you are by yourself, ALONE? Do you ever FORGET things you did while using alcohol or drugs? Do your family or FRIENDS ever tell you that you should cut down on your drinking or drug use? Have you ever gotten into TROUBLE while you were using alcohol or drugs?"

It is recommended that CRAFFT be preceded by three prescreening questions: "Have you ever drank alcohol (more than a few sips)? Have you ever smoked marijuana? Have you ever used any other drug to get high?" (17). If all three pre-screening questions are answered negatively, the CAR question (above) alone is asked. If any of the three prescreening questions is answered affirmatively, the entire CRAFFT is administered. Each positive CRAFFT response (i.e., "yes") is scored one point, and a CRAFFT total score of two or higher is considered a positive screen (16).

CRAFFT was initially validated as an oral interview, and it has subsequently been administered as a paper questionnaire. We have also developed a computerized CRAFFT screening program, which begins with the three prescreening questions, implements the appropriate skip pattern, and generates the CRAFFT total score and a printed report form for the medical care provider. What is currently unknown is which of these three administration methods adolescents might prefer. Also unknown are adolescents' preferences regarding which type of health care provider should administer the screen (nurse vs. doctor) when given as an interview, and how these administration methods might affect the adolescents' likelihood of answering the screening questions honestly.

The objective of this study was to determine adolescents' preferences for method of substance use screening with the CRAFFT, to assess how their preferences might be affected by immediate screening experiences, and how different screening methods might influence adolescents' willingness to provide honest answers. The results of this study will help health care providers to implement office systems that will yield maximal substance use screening results.

METHOD

This prospective observational study was conducted in a primary care research network that included: the Pediatric Clinic at Cambridge Hospital (Cambridge, MA); the Pediatric Practice at Fallon Clinic (Worcester, MA); the Adolescent Clinic at Tufts-New England Medical Center Floating Hospital for Children (Boston, MA); Milton Family Practice (Milton, VT); and the school-based health centers located at the Boston Community Leadership Academy (Boston, MA); Cambridge Rindge and Latin High School (Cambridge, MA); and Somerville High School (Somerville, MA). These practices reflect the wide variety of settings that provide routine health care to adolescents. They serve adolescents from urban, suburban, and rural areas, and from diverse race/ethnic and socio-economic backgrounds.

Participants were drawn from 2318 12- to 18-year-old patients arriving for routine medical care between March 2003 and August 2005. We excluded patients who were medically or emotionally unstable on the day of the medical visit (n = 10) and those who were unable to read and understand English (n = 7). Eligible patients were approached by a Research Assistant while they were in the waiting room. The Research Assistant moved those who were interested to a private area of the clinic, where she explained the purpose and procedures of the study and obtained informed assent. Over the 28-month recruitment period, 2301 patients were invited to participate and 2133 agreed (participation rate = 92.7%). Refusers (n = 168) cited as the reasons behind their decision to refuse: not wanting to be screened (n = 47), not interested in the topic (n = 44), not interested in research (n = 16), accompanied by a parent (n = 16), not enough time (n = 13), not feeling well (n = 4), other (n = 2), and no reason given (n = 26). Study participation rates did not differ significantly across practices (range 94.6% to 99.2%) except for the HMO practice, which had a significantly lower participation rate (84.3% vs. all other practices 95.5%, $p < .0001$). Eighty-two refusers gave permission for us to analyze their demographic data. Compared to participants, these refusers were more likely to be male (61.3% vs. 43.7%, $p = .003$), to be white non-Hispanic (67.1% vs. 47.9%, $p = .001$), to live with no parents or in foster care (8.0% vs. 3.0%, $p = .03$) and to be coming to the clinic for a sick visit (28.0% vs. 11.8%, $p < .0001$). However, these refusers did not differ significantly from participants in age or parent education.

The survey tool included an 8-item demographic questionnaire, a 3-item lifetime substance use questionnaire, the 6-item CRAFFT screen, and a 3-item questionnaire on participants' preferences for screening. The demographic questionnaire recorded participants age, grade in school, sex, race/ethnicity, number of parents at home, parent education level, reason for the medical visit (well care, follow-up, sick visit, other), and patient status (new patient, established patient). The 3-item lifetime substance use questionnaire separately assessed lifetime use of alcohol, marijuana, and other drugs (e.g., "Have you ever drank alcohol (more than a few sips)?").

The preferences questionnaire included one item that asked participants to rank from 1 to 4 their least preferred (1) to their most preferred (4) method of being screened for substance use. The screening administration methods to be ranked included the following: being asked questions on paper, on a computer, by a nurse, or by a doctor. A second item asked participants' to rate their comfort level with each of the same four administration methods (paper, computer, nurse, doctor) on a Likert-type response scale, where 1 = "very uncomfortable"; 2 = "a little uncomfortable"; 3 = "a little comfortable"; and 4 = "very comfortable." A third item assessed participants' likelihood of answering substance use questions honestly ("How likely are you to give completely honest answers about alcohol and drug use when asked in each of these ways?") if asked on paper, on a computer, by a nurse who knows you well, by a nurse who doesn't know you well, by a doctor who knows you well, or by a doctor who doesn't know you well (response scale for each: 1 = "very unlikely"; 2 = "a little unlikely"; 3 = "a little likely"; 4 = "very likely").

The Research Assistant read to participants the items on the demographic questionnaire, the lifetime substance use questionnaire, and the CRAFFT screen, and then entered participants' responses into a study computer. The adolescents completed the preferences questionnaire independently. A subgroup of participants (n = 222), however, completed the CRAFFT screen directly on the computer so that we could assess whether immediate experience with this mode of administration affected participants' preferences for screening and likelihood of being honest. Regardless of administration method, the RA explained to all participants that their primary care provider would receive a printed report of their responses to the CRAFFT screen. Each participant received a $2 bill after completion of the survey as compensation for his/her time. The Children's Hospital Boston Committee on Clinical Investigations and institutional review boards at each participating site approved the study protocol, including a waiver of the requirement for parental consent in accordance with published guidelines for adolescent health research (18).

Frequencies were computed for: all demographic items; any lifetime use of alcohol or drugs; CRAFFT total score, and a positive substance abuse screen ("CRAFFT+," defined as a CRAFFT total score ≥ 2). To compare CRAFFT + rates between the interview and computer groups, we used a log-Poisson model with robust error variance that was adjusted for demographic differences, because a log-binomial model did not converge (19). To compare mean ranks (for ranking item) across the different screening administration methods, we used repeated measures analysis of variance. Because the response distributions for "level of comfort" and "likelihood of honesty" were highly left-skewed, we created dichotomized variables and then used SUDAAN version 9.0 and generalized estimating equations (GEE) to compare the proportion reporting "very comfortable" or "very likely to be honest" across the different screening administration methods while controlling for demographic differences and adjusting precision estimates for sample design. To account for cluster sampling design effects, we specified clinic location and participant as nest variables, and then performed backwards selection with $p > .20$ as the exit criteria to retain only the significant demographic factors (20).

RESULTS

The study sample was 56.3% female. Distribution by age was 20.9% 12- to 13-years-old, 31.5% 14- to 16-years-old, and 47.6% 17- to 18-years-old. Composition by race/ethnicity was 48.6% white non-Hispanic, 21.9% black non-Hispanic, 10.6% Asian/Pacific islander, 8.8% Hispanic, and 11.9% other (Table 1). We included two proxy measures of socio-economic status; highest parent education level (5.3% were less than high school graduates, 40.1% completed high school or some college, and 39.1% were college graduates or higher) and number of parents living at home (63.8%

TABLE 1. Study Sample Demographic Characteristics and by Interview vs. Computer Condition

Participant Characteristics (N=2133)	All		Interview (n=1911)	Computer (n= 222)	p
	N	%	%	%	
Gender					<.0001
Female	1194	56.3	54.7	69.5	
Age					.001
13 and Under	445	20.9	21.9	12.2	
14 to 16	672	31.5	31.7	30.2	
17 Plus	1016	47.6	46.5	57.7	
Race/Ethnicity					.0001
White non-Hispanic	1022	48.6	49.9	38.0	
Black non-Hispanic	461	21.9	22.3	19.0	
Hispanic	184	8.8	8.1	14.0	
Asian/Pacific Islander	222	10.6	9.9	15.8	
Other	212	10.1	9.7	13.1	
Parents' Highest Education Level					.04
Not a High School Graduate	102	5.3	4.9	8.8	
High school grad / Some Col.	765	40.1	40.6	35.8	
College graduate / Beyond 4 years	746	39.1	38.8	41.4	
Don't know	296	15.5	15.7	14.0	
How many parents at home?					.87
One	695	33.2	33.0	34.7	
Two	1335	63.8	63.9	62.6	
None / Foster care	63	3.0	3.0	2.7	
Reason for Visit					<.0001
Well Visit / Routine	1434	67.5	70.3	42.9	
Follow-up Visit	336	15.8	14.7	25.6	
Sick Visit / Urgent Care	250	11.8	12.0	10.0	
Other	105	49.4	3.0	21.5	
Patient Status					.01
Established Patient	1957	91.7	92.3	87.4	
New Patient	176	8.3	7.7	12.6	
Substance Use					.001
Lifetime Use of alcohol and drugs	928	43.5	42.4	53.6	
CRAFFT Scores					.003
0	1391	65.3	66.6	54.8	
1	423	19.9	19.7	21.3	
2	130	6.1	5.7	10.0	
3	90	4.2	3.8	7.7	
4	47	2.2	2.1	2.7	
5	29	1.4	1.3	2.3	
6	19	0.9	0.8	1.4	
CRAFFT+ (2 or more)	315	14.8	13.7	24.0	<.0001
SITE					<.0001**
Cambridge	747	35.0	38.2	7.7	<.0001*
Fallon	483	22.6	22.9	20.3	.40*
NEMC	499	23.4	22.4	32.0	.002*
Vermont	282	13.2	13.4	11.3	.40*
Schools	122	5.7	3.0	28.8	<.0001*
**p for difference across all sites *p for difference of site vs. all others					

two parents, 33.2% one parent, 3% none/foster care). Greater than 2/3 (67.5%) of the medical visits were for routine well care and 91.7% were by established patients (i.e., not new to the practice). Overall, 43.5% of participants reported lifetime use of alcohol or drugs and 14.8% screened positive on the CRAFFT.

Compared to the group of participants who were given the CRAFFT as an interview, those who received it on the computer were more likely to be female, older, of Hispanic or Asian/Pacific Islander race/ethnicity, have parents with less education, be coming for follow-up care, to report lifetime use of alcohol or drugs, to be CRAFFT + , and to be seen at a school-based health center. We therefore controlled for these demographic factors in subsequent GEE analyses when comparing the two conditions. The odds of being CRAFFT + were significantly higher for the computer condition (OR = 1.62, 95%CI 1.10, 2.38; p = .03) compared to the interview condition. After adjusting rates for demographic differences, the computer group had a CRAFFT + rate of 19.5% vs. 13.7% for the interview group (p = .02).

Across the entire sample, paper was the screening administration method most preferred (mean rank (MR) = 2.92, 95%CI 2.87-2.96) vs. computer (MR = 2.38, 2.33-2.43), nurse (MR = 2.43, 2.39-2.47), and doctor (MR = 2.30, 2.25-2.35). Among the subgroup of participants who received the screening on the computer, however, computer (MR = 3.08, 95%CI 2.42-2.52) was statistically tied with paper (MR = 2.88, 2.75-3.02) and both were ranked significantly higher than nurse (MR = 2.06, 1.94-2.17) and doctor (MR = 1.98, 1.82-2.14).

This preference order was also supported by an analysis of the proportion of participants who responded as being "very comfortable" with these same four administration methods. For the entire sample, paper had the highest proportion "very comfortable," (74.9%) followed by computer (66.7%), doctor (59.1%), and nurse (57.0%) (Table 2).

In a GEE model that controlled for demographic factors, we found that paper yielded the highest odds of being "very comfortable" (reference), followed by computer (OR = .67, 95%CI .60-.73), and both yielded significantly higher odds than nurse (OR = .44, .39-.49) and doctor (OR = .48, .42-.54). For the subgroup of participants who experienced computer screening, however, computer was marginally higher than paper (OR = 1.4, 1.04-1.90) and substantially superior to nurse (OR = .28, .20-40) and doctor (OR = .33, .23-.47).

Because we were concerned that those who were CRAFFT + might be less comfortable with the screening process, we also performed a stratified analysis by CRAFFT screening status. We found that compared to the CRAFFT- group, those who were CRAFFT + were significantly less comfortable with all four screening administration methods, but that the order of their preferences was the same.

Across the entire sample, the highest proportion of participants (95.2%) reported being "very likely" to be honest when answering substance abuse screening questions on paper (Table 3). Statistically tied for second place were the computer (90.9%), a doctor who knows you well (90.1%), and a nurse who knows you well (88.8%). Significantly lower were a nurse who doesn't know you well (84.2%) and a doctor who doesn't know you well (83.7%). The order changes, however, when the analysis is stratified by the assessment method experienced by the participant during the study. The interview and computer condition groups differed significantly from each other across all response categories except paper. Compared to the interview condition group, those who experienced screening by computer reported greater likelihood of honesty by computer (97.7% vs. 90.1%) and lower likelihood of honesty by a nurse who doesn't know you well (72.0% vs. 85.6%), a nurse who knows you well (73.8% vs. 90.6%), a doctor who doesn't know you well (73.3% vs. 84.9%), and a doctor who knows you well (77.8% vs. 91.5%). In addition, the computer condition group showed much greater likelihood of honesty on paper and computer (96.4% and 97.7%, respectively), compared to all doctor and nurse interview categories, regardless of how well the doctor or nurse knows the adolescent (range 72.0% to 77.8%).

Perhaps even more important are the results of analysis stratified by substance abuse screening status. Among those in the CRAFFT + group, paper and computer have the highest proportions of very likely to be honest (91.1% and 88.5%, respectively), and are significantly higher than a doctor who knows you well (82.8%), a nurse who knows you well (83.1%), a doctor who doesn't know you well (79.6%), and a nurse who doesn't know you well (79.3%). The CRAFFT- group, by contast, reported significantly higher likelihood of honesty on paper (95.9%) compared to all other screening administration methods (range 84.4% to 91.3%). These findings did not change after controlling for demographic differences among subgroups.

TABLE 2. Proportion (% with 95% Confidence Interval) "Very Comfortable" with Screening Administration Method

% Participants "Very Comfortable" (N=2133)	Paper		Computer		Nurse		Doctor	
	%	p	%	p	%	p	%	p
All	74.9 (73.0, 76.7)		66.7 (64.6, 68.6)		57.0 (54.9, 59.0)		59.1 (57.0, 61.1)	
Administration Method								
Interview	76.1 (74.1, 77.9)	.001	66.0 (63.9, 68.1)	.07	59.5 (57.3, 61.7)	<.0001	61.5 (59.3, 63.6)	<.0001
Computer	65.2 (58.7, 71.1)		72.3 (66.0, 77.8)		35.0 (29.0, 41.5)		38.5 (32.3, 45.0)	
CRAFFT Scores								
CRAFFT + (2 or more)	68.1 (62.7, 73.0)	.003	61.3 (55.8, 66.6)	.03	50.3 (44.8, 55.8)	.01	51.1 (45.6, 56.6)	.002
CRAFFT -	76.1 (74.0, 78.0)		67.6 (65.4, 69.7)		58.2 (55.9, 60.4)		60.5 (58.2, 62.7)	

TABLE 3. Proportion (% with 95% Confidence Interval) Very Likely to Be Honest by Screening Administration Method

Participant Screening Scores (N=2133)	Paper		Computer		Nurse Did Not Know		Nurse Did Know		Doctor Did Not Know		Doctor Did Know	
	%	p	%	p	%	p	%	p	%	p	%	p
All	95.2 (94.2 , 96.0)		90.9 (89.6, 92.0)		84.2 (82.5, 85.7)		88.8 (87.4, 90.1)		83.7 (82.1, 85.2)		90.1 (88.8, 91.3)	
Administration Method												
Interview	95.0 (93.9, 95.9)	.51	90.1 (88.6, 91.3)	<.0001	85.6 (83.9, 87.1)	<.0001	90.6 (89.2, 91.8)	<.0001	84.9 (83.2, 86.4)	<.0001	91.5 (90.2, 92.7)	<.0001
Computer	96.4 (92.9, 98.2)		97.7 (94.7, 99.1)		72.0 (65.7, 77.5)		73.8 (67.6, 79.1)		73.3 (67.1, 78.7)		77.8 (71.9, 82.8)	
CRAFFT Scores												
CRAFFT + (2 or more)	91.1 (87.4, 93.8)	.001	88.5 (84.5, 91.6)	.136	79.3 (74.5, 83.4)	.015	83.1 (78.6, 86.9)	.001	79.6 (74.7, 83.7)	.038	82.8 (78.2, 86.6)	<.0001
CRAFFT -	95.9 (94.8, 96.7)		91.3 (89.9, 92.5)		85.0 (83.2, 86.6)		89.8 (88.3, 91.1)		84.4 (82.6, 86.0)		91.3 (90.0, 92.6)	

DISCUSSION

This study suggests that paper or computer questionnaires may be the best ways to administer substance abuse screening tests to adolescent patients in primary care medical practice. In our overall sample, paper was clearly the method with which adolescents felt most comfortable and would be most honest. In the group of participants that experienced computer screening, however, computer and paper were rated the same. It is interesting that paper and computer screening methods both provide immediate anonymity, but the participants know that the results of the screening will be given to their doctor before the forthcoming medical encounter. It may be that disclosure of behaviors that are socially proscribed, such as substance abuse, are easiest to make without an immediate face-to-face interaction. Nonetheless, some providers may find that it is easier to establish rapport with adolescent patients by using the interview method for the entire screening.

This finding may also reflect adolescents' ambivalence about engaging in alcohol and drug use. While it may be too difficult for them to acknowledge these behaviors in a personal interview, adolescents may still be worried about them. They may welcome a chance to disclose this potentially embarrassing information via a seemingly anonymous vehicle (questionnaire or computer) even though they know full well that their clinician will be given the information and question them about it further. Indeed our clinical experience suggests that this will be the case, and that one of the chief difficulties with adolescents who disclose confidential information before the medical visit, is that they may still deny the behavior during the medical encounter. Clinicians may therefore need to learn new counseling strategies to specifically deal with these conflicting responses.

Our findings are generally consistent with other studies. Turner et al. studied disclosures of confidential behavior in a sample of 1672 adolescent males randomly assigned to either paper questionnaire or computer. They found that estimates of prevalence of male-male sex, injection drug use, and sex with an injection drug user were higher by factors of 3 or more when the computer was used (21). By contrast, Vereecken et al. in a sample of more than 4000 adolescents found that administration by paper vs. computer had no significant effect on reporting of the majority of lifestyle behaviors (e.g., nutrition, leisure-time activity, sexual behavior) (22). However, there were significant differences on two of the substance use items. Among girls, there was greater disclosure of drunkenness on computer compared to paper, while among boys there was greater disclosure of hashish use on paper compared to computer.

Other studies have found computer to be generally equal to personal interviews in reliability, and superior to interviews in reporting of stigmatized behaviors as evidenced by higher prevalence rates (23,24). We found a higher prevalence of CRAFFT + results in our computer condition compared to the interview, even after controlling for demographic differences. This result should be viewed cautiously, however, because our conditions were not randomly assigned. In addition, no studies have yet assessed the interrater reliability of the CRAFFT, nor has the validity of the CRAFFT been assessed when administered by different methods (e.g., paper vs. computer vs. interview).

This study had a number of strengths. It was conducted in a variety of practice types and locations, and the sample size was moderately large. It used a well-validated screening test, the CRAFFT, and we received a waiver of the requirement for parental consent, minimizing the likelihood of self-selection bias. This study also has potential limitations. It was conducted in practices in New England only. Other regions of the country may be different. The survey relied on adolescents' self report to measure substance use. However, previous studies have shown self-report to be a reliable means of measuring substance use and it compares favorably with other methods of substance use detection–such as laboratory testing (25).

Nonetheless, our findings indicate that either paper or computer-based confidential questionnaires can be used to screen adolescent primary care patients for substance use, both those patients who are likely to screen negative and those likely to screen positive. Given the large number of risk and problem behaviors for which providers should screen and the time constraints in their schedules, inexpensive and easy to score multi-problem questionnaires need to be developed that include the CRAFFT substance abuse screen and other validated instruments that screen for other risk behaviors.

Our findings have other implications for adolescent medical practice. First, providers will need to further assess those adolescents who screen positive for substance use problems. Given the time constraints of office visits, it may be necessary to ask screen-positive teens to return to the office for a separate appointment so that an adequate alcohol and drug assessment can be completed. Providers will need training in implementation of brief advice and counseling techniques for adolescents with problematic use and abuse, and they need to be able to make timely referrals to more intensive treatment programs for adolescent patients who are diagnosed with alcohol or drug dependence. More research is needed on efficient and effective office-based systems for substance abuse screening and therapeutic interventions.

REFERENCES

1. Johnston LD, O'Malley PM, Bachman JG, et al: Monitoring the future national results on adolescent drug use: Overview of key findings, 2005 (NIH Publication No. 06-5882), in. Bethesda, MD: National Institute on Drug Abuse, 2006.

2. Eaton DK, Kann L, Kinchen SA, et al.: Youth Risk Behavior Surveillance–United States, 2005. MMWR 55:SS-5, 2006.

3. Hingson RW, Heeren T, Winter MR: Age at drinking onset and alcohol dependence: age at onset, duration, and severity. Arch Pediatr Adolesc Med 160: 739, 2006.

4. Burge V, Felts M, Chenier T, et al.: Drug use, sexual activity, and suicidal behavior in U.S. high school students. Journal of School Health. 65:222, 1995.

5. DuRant R, Knight J, Goodman E: Factors associated with aggressive and delinquent behaviors among patients attending an adolescent medicine clinic. J Adolesc Health 21:303, 1997.

6. DuRant RH, Smith JA, Kreiter SR, et al.: The relationship between early age of onset of initial substance use and engaging in multiple health risk behaviors among young adolescents. Arch Pediatr Adolesc Med 153:286, 1999.

7. Patton GC, Coffey C, Carlin JB, et al.: Cannabis use and mental health in young people: cohort study. BMJ 325:1195, 2002.

8. Knight JR: The role of the primary care provider in preventing and treating alcohol problems in adolescents. Ambulatory Pediatrics. 1:150, 2001.

9. Kulig JW: Tobacco, alcohol, and other drugs: the role of the pediatrician in prevention, identification, and management of substance abuse. Pediatrics 115:816, 2005.

10. Vaughan BL, Levy S, Knight JR: Adolescent substance abuse: Prevention and management by primary care clinicians. Journal of Clinical Outcomes Management 10:166, 2003.

11. Green M, Palfrey J (eds.): Bright Futures: Guidelines for Health Supervision of Infants, Children, and Adolescents, 2nd Edition), Arlington, VA: National Center for Education in Maternal and Child Health, 2000.

12. Knight J, Shrier L, Bravender T, et al.: A new brief screen for adolescent substance abuse. Arch Pediatr Adolesc Med 153:591, 1999.

13. Rahdert ER (ed): The Adolescent Assessment/Referral System Manual, ed DHHS Publication No. (ADM)91-1735): US Dept Health Human Services (PHS) Alcohol, Drug Abuse, and Mental Health Administration, 1991.

14. Babor T, de la Fuente J, Saunders J, et al.: AUDIT: The Alcohol Use Disorders Identification Test: Guidelines for use in primary health care, Geneva, Switzerland: World Health Organization, 1992.

15. Knight JR, Sherritt L, Harris SK, et al.: Validity of brief alcohol screening tests among adolescents: A comparison of the AUDIT, POSIT, CAGE and CRAFFT. Alcohol Clin Exp Res 27:67, 2002.

16. Knight JR, Sherritt L, Shrier LA, et al.: Validity of the CRAFFT substance abuse screening test among adolescent clinic patients. Arch Pediatr Adolesc Med 156:607, 2002.

17. Levy S, Knight JR: Office management of substance use. Adolescent Health Update 15:1, 2003.

18. Society for Adolescent Medicine: Guidelines for adolescent health research. J Adolesc Health 17:264, 1995.

19. Zou G: A modified poisson regression approach to prospective studies with binary data. Am J Epidemiol 159:702, 2004.

20. Mickey RM, Greenland S: The impact of confounder selection criteria on effect estimation. Am J Epidemiology 129:125, 1989.

21. Turner CF, Ku L, Rogers SM, et al.: Adolescent sexual behavior, drug use, and violence: increased reporting with computer survey technology. Science. 280:867, 1998.

22. Vereecken CA, Maes L: Comparison of a computer-administered and paper- and-pencil-administered questionnaire on health and lifestyle behaviors. J Adolesc Health 38:426, 2006.

23. Williams ML, Freeman RC, Bowen AM, et al.: A comparison of the reliability of self-reported drug use and sexual behaviors using computer-assisted versus face-to-face interviewing (and other abstracts) AIDS Educ Prev. 12:199, 2000

24. van Griensven F, Naorat S, Kilmarx PH, et al.: Palmtop-assisted self-interviewing for the collection of sensitive behavioral data: randomized trial with drug use urine testing. Am J Epidemiol 163:271, 2006.

25. Murphy DA, Durako S, Muenz LR, et al.: Marijuana use among HIV-positive and high-risk adolescents: a comparison of self-report through audio computer-assisted self-administered interviewing and urinalysis. Am J Epidemiol 152:805, 2000.

doi:10.1300/J465v28n04_03

"No-Contact" Interventions for Unhealthy College Drinking: Efficacy of Alternatives to Person-Delivered Intervention Approaches

Rebecca N. Zisserson, MA
Tibor P. Palfai, PhD
Richard Saitz, MD, MPH

SUMMARY. Despite the development of brief efficacious interventions, they are not reaching a large proportion of college students who continue to drink in a manner that puts them at risk for harm. Recent efforts have attempted to address this issue through the development of brief alcohol interventions that may be more broadly disseminated to college students. Researchers have adapted a variety of approaches to print and computer-based modalities that do not require direct real-time contact with an interventionist. The goal of this paper is to review the empirical evidence for the utility of these brief alcohol interventions that are delivered without direct real-time contact. A systematic review of this research suggests that "no-contact" interventions are feasible and may have efficacy. Further research is needed to understand the duration of these effects, mechanisms of change, moderators of outcome, and how to enhance the effectiveness of these approaches. doi:10.1300/J465v28n04_04 *[Article copies available for a fee from The Haworth Document Delivery Service: 1-800-HAWORTH. E-mail address: <docdelivery@haworthpress.com> Website: <http://www.HaworthPress.com> © 2007 by The Haworth Press, Inc. All rights reserved.]*

KEYWORDS. No-contact, alcohol, college students, brief interventions, internet

Unhealthy alcohol use (1) (excessive drinking, alcohol abuse and dependence) on college campuses is prevalent and causes substantial harm. Forty-four percent of college students report heavy episodic drinking (also known as binge drinking, defined as 4 or more drinks for women and 5 or more for men on an occasion), and these students have a higher risk of alco-

Rebecca N. Zisserson and Tibor P. Palfai are affiliated with the Department of Psychology, Boston University, Boston, MA.

Richard Saitz is affiliated with the Clinical Addiction Research and Education (CARE) Unit, Section of General Internal Medicine, Boston University School of Medicine and Boston Medical Center, Boston, MA, and Department of Epidemiology and the Youth Alcohol Prevention Center, Boston University School of Public Health, Boston, MA.

Address correspondence to: Rebecca N. Zisserson, MA, Department of Psychology, Boston University, 648 Beacon Street, 4th Floor, Boston, MA 02215 (E-mail: rebeccaz@bu.edu).

[Haworth co-indexing entry note]: " 'No-Contact' Interventions for Unhealthy College Drinking: Efficacy of Alternatives to Person-Delivered Intervention Approaches." Zisserson, Rebecca N., Tibor P. Palfai, and Richard Saitz. Co-published simultaneously in *Substance Abuse* (The Haworth Medical Press, an imprint of The Haworth Press, Inc.) Vol. 28, No. 4, 2007, pp. 119-131; and: *Alcohol/Drug Screening and Brief Intervention: Advances in Evidence-Based Practice* (ed: Richard Saitz, and Marc Galanter) The Haworth Medical Press, an imprint of The Haworth Press, Inc., 2007, pp. 119-131. Single or multiple copies of this article are available for a fee from The Haworth Document Delivery Service [1-800-HAWORTH, 9:00 a.m. - 5:00 p.m. (EST). E-mail address: docdelivery@haworthpress.com].

Available online at http://suba.haworthpress.com

doi:10.1300/J465v28n04_04

hol-related problems such as alcohol poisoning, serious injury, assault, and academic problems (2-4). Past-year prevalence of alcohol abuse and dependence in college students is 31% and 6%, respectively (5). Furthermore, students are affected by other students' heavy drinking in the form of unwanted sexual advances, assaults, and disruptions in studying (3,4).

A number of individual interventions have been developed to address unhealthy alcohol use by college students. The most efficacious of these interventions are individually-focused cognitive-behavioral skills-training and brief motivational interventions (6). Effective cognitive-behavioral skills training interventions, which focus on teaching skills to modify beliefs or behaviors associated with drinking, include alcohol expectancy challenges (7,8), self-monitoring (9,10), and alcohol skills training programs (ASTP), comprised of information on how to limit drinking, blood alcohol concentration (BAC) discrimination, and assertiveness and drink-refusal skills (10-12). There is also strong support for brief motivational interventions, which are one to two session interviews designed to increase motivation to change drinking, and generally include personalized normative feedback (PNF) on drinking behavior, skills-training information, and advice on how to reduce drinking (13-15).

Although these interventions have proven efficacy, they are not reaching large numbers of students with unhealthy alcohol use. Few students are screened for unhealthy alcohol use, and the majority of students are not interested in participating in traditional alcohol programs (16-18). Recently, there has been evidence that interventions can be useful in decreasing unhealthy alcohol use even if they are not delivered by a person (e.g., counselor or interventionist). These "no-contact" interventions include mailed information about alcohol use patterns and consequences and computer/web-based approaches. Efforts to promote change in alcohol use without the need for contact with an interventionist have a number of advantages. First, these methods are able to reach a larger number of students than traditional individual or group interventions. For example, in 2002 over half of the U.S. population had internet access at home (19), and 93% of college students regularly use the internet (20). Second, these interventions might be appealing to a wider range of people, particularly those that would not participate in more intensive treatments because of fear of labeling, lack of time, or belief that the problem is not that serious (21). A third advantage is the cost of these approaches: for example, effective mailed feedback interventions cost about two dollars per student (22). Finally, these approaches may facilitate the delivery of longer-term or more extensive interventions without the cost and time of therapist contact. With continued concerns about the high relapse rates among those who are exposed to health change interventions (23), these no-contact interventions provide an opportunity to support changes in alcohol use over time with minimal time requirements for the individual (24).

Researchers have recently demonstrated the feasibility of using no-contact interventions among a variety of populations. There is a wide age and geographic representation of people who are already using internet sites for recovery from substance abuse and dependence (25), and there is some demand in the general population for internet screening (26-28). Evidence suggests that people in the general population as well as college students find anonymous web-based personalized feedback more appealing than practitioner-delivered interventions (29,30). Although no-contact computer-based interventions are being used by hundreds of colleges and universities, little is known regarding their efficacy (31). Given preliminary evidence of their feasibility, interest, and low-cost, and their current use without sufficient research, it is important to review what we know about these approaches. The goal of this paper is to review the extant literature on the empirical support for no-contact interventions for reducing unhealthy drinking among college students.

METHODS

To review the research on no-contact interventions, we used three sources: (1) database searches of MEDLINE and PsychINFO using the terms *internet*, *computer*, *mailed*, *bibliotherapy*, and *intervention*, combined with *college*, *university*, *alcohol*, *and drinking*, (2) reference lists in published papers on alcohol intervention studies or on websites of the internet interventions, (3) proceedings of scientific conferences. Studies were included in this review if: (1) subjects were college students, (2) there was at least one intervention condition in the study that did not involve direct real-time contact and one comparison condition, and (3) the study reported at least one outcome related to alcohol consumption or alcohol consequences. Studies that met the above criteria but included extensive in person contact were excluded. Only published studies are included in this review. While these interventions are designed to target unhealthy alcohol users, this review is not limited to studies that screened participants for unhealthy alcohol use.

RESULTS

Fourteen studies were identified that met inclusion criteria, but 3 were excluded because in addition to the no contact intervention there was substantial in-person contact (32-34). Therefore, a total of 11 studies are included in this review, and Table 1 summarizes the results of these studies. Ten of these studies showed some efficacy for no-contact interventions for unhealthy alcohol use. The number of participants ranged from 26 to 2,194, and the length of follow-up assessments ranged from one month to twelve months. The studies that met our review criteria fell into two categories of interventions: mailed interventions and computer-based interventions.

Mailed Interventions

In 6 studies the intervention was mailed to the participants. In a pilot study, Agostinelli and colleagues (35) studied mailing a PNF pamphlet based on the Drinker's Check-Up (DCU) (36). Of 568 psychology students screened, 64 heavy drinkers, defined by consuming at least 80 drinks in the past month, were identified. Twenty-six students accepted the offer to participate in a research study and were randomly assigned to receive or not receive a mailed intervention. The feedback included information on weekly average drinks compared to the U.S. population according to gender, as well as peak BAC levels, tolerance, and family history. Six weeks after the mailing, all but three participants returned for an in-person follow up interview. Compared to the control group, those who received the intervention decreased weekly drinks and average weekly peak BAC, but not highest peak BAC, which remained elevated in both groups.

As cited in Saunders et al. (37), Laforge and colleagues also studied the effect of a mailed feedback intervention. After screening a random sample of 1,638 matriculating students, 1,067 students who drank two or more drinks on one occasion at any time in the past year and did not exhibit signs of alcohol dependence were randomly assigned to receive a feedback report or assessments only. Feedback reports were mailed after baseline, 3-months, and 6-months, and were tailored to the individual by a computer program that selected intervention messages based on the individuals' frequency of high risk drinking, readiness to change, and situational temptations. The reports included information on the participants' comparative risk, behavioral and cognitive practices, and self-help information, and the follow-up mailings included feedback about progress toward change. Eighty percent of subjects completed the 3- and 6-month follow-ups, and 77% completed the 12-month. Treatment effectiveness was moderated by gender: for women, the intervention decreased alcohol problems and high-risk alcohol behaviors (e.g., heavy episodic drinking) at 3 months, and the difference was sustained at 6 and 12 months compared to the control group. There were no significant intervention effects for men.

Collins and colleagues (38) recruited 100 students reporting at least two heavy drinking episodes in the past month through psychology classes, and randomized students, stratified on gender, to a mailed PNF group or a control group. The 2-page mailed PNF included information on the frequency and quantity of drinking, frequency of heavy drinking episodes, typical peak BAC, alcohol-related problems, U.S. and university-specific normative drinking information, and didactic material on BAC, tolerance, and heavy drinking to help explain the feedback. The control group received a psychoeducational brochure on alcohol use. Sub-

TABLE 1. Studies with Comparison Groups of No-Contact Interventions for Unhealthy College Drinking

Study	N	Recruitment	Study Groups	Outcome Measures	Results
Mailed interventions					
Agostinelli et al., 1995	26	Psychology classes	Mailed PNF Assessment only	weekly drinks, average weekly peak BAC, highest peak BAC	6 week: PNF decreased weekly drinks, average weekly peak BAC
Saunders et al., 2004	1067	Screened via telephone from random list	3 mailed PNFs Assessment only	composite score of high-risk alcohol consumption, alcohol problems	3 month, 6 month, 12 month: PNF decreased high-risk alcohol consumption and problems for women only
Collins et al., 2002	100	Psychology classes	Mailed PNF Psychoeducation brochure	drinks/heaviest drinking week, # heavy drinking episodes, peak BAC, alcohol problems	6 week: PNF decrease drinks/heaviest drinking week, # heavy drinking episodes 6 month: not significant
Walters et al., 2000	43	Psychology classes	Mailed PNF only Mailed PNF + 2-hour group intervention Assessment only	drinks/month, peak wkly and monthly BAC, alcohol expectancies, alcohol problems	6 week: PNF only differed from the control group in decrease of drinks/month
Walters, 2000	46	Psychology classes	Mailed PNF only 2-hour group intervention with PNF Assessment only	drinks/week	6 week: PNF only had largest decrease in drinks/week
Johnsson & Berglund, 2005	177	Freshman orientation	Mailed PNF only 5 two-hour ASTP groups + PNF	AUDIT	1 year: both groups significantly decreased AUDIT scores; no group differences
Computer-based interventions					
Kypri et al., 2004	104	University health center	On-site web PNF Web assessment + pamphlet	total # drinks, # heavy drinking episodes, alcohol problems, # drinking days, # drinks/typical occasion, academic consequences	6 week: PNF decreased # drinks, heavy drinking episodes, alcohol problems 6 month: PNF decreased alcohol problems
Neighbors et al., 2004	252	Psychology classes	On-site web PNF Web assessment only	drinking behavior, perceived norms	3 month, 6 month: PNF had greater reductions in drinking and perceived norms
Chiauzzi et al., 2005	265	Newspaper ads, fliers	Off-site 4-session web-based PNF Off-site 4-session informational website	max drinks/day, drinking composite score, special occasion consumption, alcohol problems, average # binge episodes, drinks/week, drinking days/week, average drinks/drinking day	post-intervention: web PNF had greater reductions in max drinks/day than control 3 month: web PNF delayed the increase in drinking, greater decrease in special occasion consumption for women, fewer alcohol problems for women
Moore et al., 2005	116	3 college courses	4 off-site web-based alcohol newsletters 4 mailed alcohol newsletters	1-year frequency, 2-week binge-drinking frequency, 30-day frequency, quantity, binge-drinking frequency, "get drunk" frequency, "get drunk" quantity, greatest number of drinks	30-day: both groups reduced 30-day frequency; no differences between groups
Saitz et al., 2007	2194	E-mail	Off-site web-based minimal PNF Off-site web-based extensive PNF	Readiness to Change (RTC), AUDIT, drinks/week, heavy drinking episodes, max drinks per occasion	Post-intervention: Men in the extensive PNF condition were more likely to report intention to seek help. Women in the extensive PNF had a greater increase in RTC. 1 month: No group differences.

jects received course credit for completing the 6-week post-test and $10 for completing the 6-month follow-up. Ninety-four percent of subjects returned for the 6-week assessment, and 65% returned after 6 months. At the 6-week follow-up, the intervention group was drinking significantly less than the control group as measured by drinks per heaviest drinking week and number of heavy drinking episodes, but no effect was found between groups in alcohol problems or peak BAC. No significant effects were found at the 6-month follow up, nor were interaction effects of gender and group at either time point. Finally, although after the intervention those in the PNF group had a higher perceived discrepancy between their drinking and their peers' drinking (normative discrepancy) than the control group, the data did not support normative discrepancy as playing a mediational role.

Walters et al. (39) compared a mailed feedback intervention to no intervention and a mailed intervention plus a brief group alcohol intervention. Forty-three heavy drinking students, defined by consuming at least 40 drinks in the past month, were recruited from psychology classes and were randomly assigned to one of three groups. A Feedback Only (FBO) group received a mailed PNF based on the DCU, which included information about quantity and frequency of drinking per week and per month, comparison to national and campus norms by converting to a percentile, peak weekly and monthly BAC levels, money spent on alcohol per year and percent of income spent on alcohol, and level of tolerance. A Full Treatment (FT) group participated in a 2-hour group intervention providing educational, attitudinal, and skills-based techniques to promote moderation and responsible decision making when drinking, and included a drinking norms clarification exercise. The FT group also received the same mailed PNF one week later. The control group received no intervention. Eighty-six percent of students returned for the 6-week follow-up assessment. While the two intervention groups had decreases in drinks per month, only the FBO group significantly differed from the control group. There were no significant differences between groups in peak weekly or monthly BAC levels, and there were no significant effects on alcohol expectancies or alcohol problems. Surprisingly, the group intervention might have detracted from the effectiveness of the mailed feedback. The authors suggest that one reason for this might be that being with other heavy drinkers had a normalizing effect on one's drinking behavior, thereby undermining the messages in the norm-correcting personalized feedback. Another possible reason for this effect may be that the FBO group read the feedback more carefully than the FT group, who received the feedback after the class. To address this issue, Walters (22) conducted another study comparing FBO, FT and no intervention, in which FT included a 2-hour group intervention that integrated PNF but did not include a mailing. Forty-six students were randomly assigned, and 34 subjects returned for the 6-week follow-up. The participants in the FBO condition again had the largest decrease in drinks per week compared to the other two groups.

Johnsson and Berglund (40) also evaluated a mailed PNF in comparison to a group intervention, but here the group intervention was a more extensive 10-hour Alcohol Skills Training Program (ASTP). Six hundred and ninety-three freshman orientation students were asked to participate in the study and screened during the orientation. One-hundred seventy-seven hazardous drinkers, defined as scoring in the highest quartile on the Alcohol Use Disorders Identification Test (AUDIT) (41), were randomly assigned to receive a mailed PNF or an ASTP. The PNF consisted of feedback that the students were in the upper quartile of AUDIT scores of the students they screened, recommendations to drink less and if necessary seek professional help. In addition to the same AUDIT-based PNF the PNF group received, the students in the ASTP group participated in five weekly two-hour groups at the student health center. Each group was lead by a member of the research team and two trained peer "co-educators." The program was based on the Brief Alcohol Screening and Intervention for College Students (BASICS) (42) manual, and included feedback on AUDIT scores, facts and myths about alcohol, a discussion on gender roles, an alcohol expectancy challenge, and planning for high-risk drinking situations. Students self-monitored their alcohol consumption for the duration of the course for discussion. Follow-up questionnaires were mailed to all participants one year after baseline, 84% of whom responded. After one year, both groups had significantly decreased AUDIT scores, though there were no significant differences between the groups in total AUDIT scores.

Computer-Based Interventions

Computer-based interventions are those computer program or internet interventions where the intervention takes place in either a controlled setting, such as a hospital or school facility, "on-site," or at a computer of the participant's choice (at home, in a computer lab, etc.), "off-site." Computer-based interventions with community samples have been found to reduce alcohol consumption for up to one year (43,44).

There have been five studies evaluating the efficacy of computer-based interventions with college students. In the first on-site intervention, Kypri and colleagues (45) screened 167 students visiting a health center for unhealthy alcohol use, defined by a score of 8 or more on the AUDIT (41) and the consumption of more than four (for women) or six (for men) standard drinks on at least one occasion in the past month. One hundred and four students meeting criteria were randomized to either a web-based PNF intervention or a control group. The program consisted of assessment of drinking and perceptions of peer drinking norms followed by a summary of recent consumption, risk status, comparison of their consumption with recommended limits, highest BAC and health effects on the body, comparison of drinking with national and university norms, correction of norm misperceptions, and information on how to get help if concerned (http://ipru.otago.ac.nz/sbi1demo/login.html). The control group received an identical assessment and was given an alcohol information pamphlet. Six weeks after the intervention, participants were e-mailed a link to the follow-up website along with a lunch voucher, and 6 months after the intervention participants were mailed a paper-and-pencil questionnaire. Six-week follow-up data were obtained from 80% of participants, and 6-month data was obtained from 90% of participants. At 6 weeks, compared to controls, the intervention resulted in reduced total number of drinks, number of heavy drinking episodes, and alcohol-related problems. No significant differences were found for number of drinking days, number of drinks per typical occasion, or consequences relating to academic performance. At 6 months, reductions in consumption were no longer significant but reductions in alcohol-related problems were significantly greater in the intervention group.

Neighbors and colleagues (46) conducted a similar on-site assessment of a computer-based intervention. Yet unlike previous no-contact interventions, this intervention included only PNF on frequency and quantity of alcohol consumption, without additional intervention components such as risk factors. Students were screened from a sample of 1,115 students from psychology classes, and a total of 252 students expressing interest in the study and reporting at least one heavy drinking episode in the previous month were recruited. Subjects were given extra course credit for baseline assessments, $15 for the 3-month follow-up, and $25 for the 6-month follow-up. All students were given computerized assessments in a controlled setting on-campus, including measures of perceived drinking norms, social motives, expectancies, and evaluations of the social effects of alcohol. Individuals randomly assigned to the intervention group immediately received PNF, modeled after the feedback component of BASICS (42) that included a summary of the subjects' perceived drinking norms and actual drinking norms at their college. The feedback was viewed on the computer screen for one minute and was printed out for the subject to take home. Compared to the control group at both 3 and 6 months, the intervention group had greater reductions in drinking and perceived norms, and changes in perceived norms at 3 months mediated consumption effects at 6 months. Neighbors et al. (46) also examined social motives for drinking, an individual difference factor directly related to the content of the intervention. Students in the intervention group who had social motives for drinking had greater reduction in drinking than others at 3 months, but not at 6 months.

While the previous two computer-based interventions took place on-site, Chiauzzi and colleagues (47) were the first to publish a study on an off-site computerized intervention. The authors evaluated an internet-based brief intervention called My Student Body (MSB), which has alcohol, tobacco, and sexually transmitted diseases versions (mystudentbody.com). While screening and orientation took place on-site and with a research assistant, the intervention took place off-site, at the participants' personal computers via the internet. Of the 538 students at 5 universities who were recruited through college newspaper ads, flyers, and recruitment tables, 265 students who had at least one heavy drinking episode in the past week were randomized to the MSB intervention website or a control website. Students were compensated $5 for the screening and $135 for attending an orientation session and completing assessments. MSB is based on BASICS and focuses on the students' beliefs about alcohol, lifestyle issues, risks they take while drinking, and alcohol-related consequences. The site also includes information on drinking-related risks, how to help another student who is drinking too much, health news, social norm information, moderate drinking strategies, and peer stories. The control website, Alcohol and You, had articles on the effects of drinking and did not include any interactive or motivational elements. Participants could access the websites from any computer with a personal log-in code, for four weekly 20-minute sessions. Twenty percent of students either dropped out of the study or were lost to follow-up. MSB intervention students had greater immediate post-intervention (one-month after baseline) reductions in maximum drinks per day than the control group, but by 3-months, both groups reported similar maximums. Although both groups increased drinking by the 3-month follow-up, MSB delayed this increase, based on a composite score that consisted of past-week consumption, average number of binge episodes, and maximum drinks per drinking day. At the 3-month follow-up, women in the MSB group showed significantly greater reductions in total consumption during special occasions than women in the control group, and women in the MSB group reported significantly fewer alcohol-related problems than women in the control group. Significant results were not found for average number of heavy drinking episodes, drinks per week, drinking days per week, and average drinks per drinking day. Among the subgroup of students who continued to drink heavily at the 3-month follow-up ("persistent heavy drinkers"), those who received the MSB experienced a more rapid decrease in average and peak consumption as well as in the alcohol composite score from baseline to immediately post-intervention, and effects were maintained at follow-up. There were no group differences in readiness to change over time, although drinkers low in motivation to change in the intervention group reduced average consumption at a faster rate than low-motivation drinkers in the control group. Therefore the MSB intervention seemed particularly useful for persistent heavy drinkers, women, and low-motivation drinkers.

Moore and colleagues (48) evaluated a second off-site computerized intervention. In order to determine whether or not internet-based interventions are as efficacious as mailed interventions, the authors compared a web-based intervention to an identical mailed print-based version. Participants were recruited from three college courses regardless of drinking status, and one hundred sixteen students filled out online baseline questionnaires and were randomized to one of the two conditions. Three weeks after baseline questionnaires were completed, the students were either e-mailed or post-mailed four newsletters at one-week intervals. Thirty days after completing the intervention, students were e-mailed a link to an online follow-up questionnaire, with 86% of students responding. Students received extra credit for their courses as well as received $5 for completing each of two surveys. The intervention was based on the Extended Parallel Process Model (EPPM) (49) and included challenging alcohol-expectancies, definitions of standard drinks and binge drinking, strategies to reduce binge drinking, and internet links to alcohol information and services. At the 30-day follow-up, the web-based and print-based groups did not differ on past-year frequency, 30-day frequency, 30-day quantity, 30-day binge-drinking frequency, 30-day "get drunk" frequency, 30-day "get drunk" quantity, 30-day greatest number of drinks, or 2-week binge-drinking frequency. For all participants regardless of group, past 30-day frequency was significantly reduced. To examine if either type of intervention was more efficacious for specific groups of students, the authors conducted a secondary analysis using assignment by binge status and gender. There were no significant interactions for assignment by binge or gender. However, a binge by time interaction was significant, with binge drinkers experiencing a decrease in 30-day average quantity, drink quantity, and greatest number of drinks, while non binge-drinkers increased their drinking on these variables.

Finally, Saitz et al. (50) conducted a study that utilized the internet for recruitment, intervention, and follow-up assessments. The study assessed recruitment strategies for online alcohol screening for the entire freshman class at a large urban university, as well as pilot tested two versions of a brief internet intervention. All freshman students who were at least 18 years old and had a valid university e-mail address were randomized to receive either an invitation with a hyperlink to a general health screening, or to an alcohol-specific screening. After the assessment, students with AUDIT scores of 8 or above were randomized to receive either additional information ("extensive" intervention) or no additional information ("minimal" intervention). Both interventions included gender-specific graphic comparisons to local norms for drinks per week and number of heavy drinking episodes, as well as information about drinking guidelines. The extensive intervention included additional feedback on highest blood alcohol level, a personalized graphic profile of negative consequences of drinking experienced in the past year with gender-specific normative information of the percent of freshman experiencing these consequences, feedback on the amount of money spent per week and per year on alcohol, the number of calories from alcohol consumed per month, and time on a treadmill required to burn those calories to maintain current weight. The intervention was followed by additional assessments and an invitation to receive a follow-up survey one month later, the completion of which would enter them into a drawing for a $100 Amazon.com gift certificate or an Apple iPod. One month later, students who enrolled in the follow-up received an e-mail to complete a final assessment. Of 4,008 freshman students e-mailed, 2,194 (54.7%) completed the initial assessment. There were no significant differences in completion rate between the general health invitation group and the alcohol-specific invitation group. Immediately post-intervention, only men in the extensive intervention group were more likely to report intention to seek help than men in the minimal intervention group. For women only, those in the extensive intervention group had a significantly greater increase in their readiness to change compared to those in the minimal intervention group. Seventy-five percent of students completed the one-month follow-up. Across both intervention groups, women significantly decreased drinks per week and heavy drinking episodes, while a decrease in maximum drinks per occasion was not significant. There were no changes in consumption among males. There were no significant differences in outcome variables between the minimal and extensive intervention groups.

COMMENT

Mailed and computer-based no-contact interventions are promising ways to reduce alcohol use among college students. Given the prevalence of unhealthy alcohol use among college students and the difficulty of engaging students in treatment, alcohol interventions that are disseminated to all students and are easily, quickly, and anonymously completed seem particularly important to further explore in this population. These types of interventions also provide considerable flexibility in terms of content and links with other information. Findings from the mailed feedback and computer-based studies indicate these interventions can decrease college student alcohol consumption and last at least 6 weeks after the intervention is delivered, though evidence for longer-lasting effects and reductions in alcohol problems is less clear.

There are already a number of ongoing and unpublished studies of computerized feedback interventions that indicate no-contact interventions are effective at reducing short-term drinking (51-54). What is most encouraging about the results from controlled studies of no-contact interventions is that the effect of these interventions on drinking behavior is comparable to the effect of in-person interventions of similar content. For example, the within-group effect size for the intervention group for the in-person brief intervention based on the DCU was 0.33 (36), while the within-group effect sizes for consumption measures for the no-contact mailed feedback interventions based on the DCU were 0.68 (35), 1.01 (39), and 0.63 (22). Hester and Delaney (43) found that with adults, the within-group effect size of a computerized behavioral self control training program was 1.04, on par with average effect sizes of 1.11 for in-person or therapist-assisted self-help versions of behavioral self control training (55). Finally, the between-group effect sizes for the Kypri and colleagues' (45) computer-based feedback intervention for college students are comparable to those reported in a meta-analysis of brief interventions in the general population (56).

Furthermore, the addition of in-person counseling does not appear to improve the efficacy of no-contact interventions (22,39,40). Murphy et al. (32) and White and colleagues (34) found that discussing personalized feedback with a counselor did not increase the intervention's efficacy over simply handing the feedback to the participant without a discussion. Indeed, some research has shown that the addition of an in-person intervention to a mailed feedback may detract from the efficacy of the feedback-based intervention (22,39).

Despite the overall promising findings, there are methodological characteristics common to these studies that need to be considered in interpreting the results. First, the recruitment strategies may limit the generalizability of the results. College students have been typically recruited through psychology classes, and researchers used course credit and/or money as incentives for completion of the interventions. If such interventions are going to be broadly disseminated and utilized, it may be beneficial to examine approaches that will more closely approximate the ways that populations will ultimately be targeted, such as freshmen orientation sessions. Also, considering the pervasive use of the internet by college students, expanding recruitment procedures to include university-wide e-mails and links on frequently visited websites may also be a useful means to explore. Saitz and colleagues (50) have already demonstrated the feasibility of such recruitment techniques and the promising rate of responding students.

Second, most studies use assessment-only control conditions, which do not control for possible effects of time spent reading about alcohol or other non-specific factors. Control conditions that are approximately the same form and length as the intervention, similar to Chiauzzi and colleagues' (47) Alcohol and You website condition, would help to clarify the meaning of the effects of the interventions. Kypri and colleagues (45) found evidence that multiple assessments may contribute to decreases in drinking at 6-month follow-ups, and including control conditions in further studies that do not have one of the assessments would help in determining whether or not the baseline or first follow-up assessments have a beneficial impact. Also, three studies did not have a true control group at all, making it difficult to determine the impact of the no-contact intervention alone (40,48,50).

None of the efficacy studies on the feedback-based no-contact interventions with students assessed the extent to which the participants identified the feedback as accurately portraying their drinking. Results with adults in the community suggest that feedback may not be perceived as accurate if the subjects' drinking is not regular (27), and attention should be given to the form of feedback presented. Given that one hypothesized mechanism of change is the recognition that one's drinking is deviating from what is normal, it would be important to assess the extent to which the students feel like both information about the drinking of others and feedback on their own drinking is accurate and relevant to their behavior.

Three of the computer-based interventions took place off-site instead of in a laboratory or health setting. Although researchers are currently investigating other off-site computer-based interventions, notably the PNF-based website www.e-chug.com (54), in two of these studies the intervention itself is completed at home, but there is still contact with the researcher in the form of orientation sessions, phone calls, or baseline and follow-up assessments. Intervention strategies similar to those used by Saitz et al. (50) where all therapist and researcher contact is eliminated and students are mailed or e-mailed recruitment information, assessment, intervention, and follow-up questionnaires should continue to be investigated.

Although research on no-contact interventions for college students has been promising, there are many remaining issues, including moderators of treatment effects, duration of the effects, optimal content of the interventions, and other new technologies that might be utilized. One of the main issues is whether these interventions are differentially effective for different students. Studies on the moderating effects of gender, for example, suggest that feedback may be more effective for women (37,47). Chiauzzi and colleagues (47) also found that their intervention was effective only for heavier drinkers, and Moore et al. (48) found that the internet and mailed interventions were effective for binge drinkers and not for non-binge drinkers. Results from an adult population suggest that the extent to which one perceives his or herself to be at risk for alcohol-related harm may affect the efficacy of the intervention (57), and Walters and Woodall (58) found increases in perceived risk mediated changes in drinking. Because college students do not always agree with administrators and researchers on definitions of risky alcohol use and many students are reluctant to label dangerous behaviors associated with drinking as indicating a problem (59), when constructing no-contact interventions the role of perceived risk may be an important variable to assess.

Drinking motives have been identified as important factors that may differentiate responses to interventions (60). One study (46) found evidence that PNF interventions may be more effective with students who have social motives for drinking. Because the only component of their intervention was PNF, which relies on the assumption that students value how much they are drinking compared to their peers, this finding is not surprising. However, it would be beneficial to understand how drinking motives affect the efficacy of no-contact interventions in general, and if there might be ways to include aspects of PNF interventions that specifically target students who drink to cope with negative affect, for example. Further research in what works for whom could lead to better-tailored interventions.

Other important questions remain about the content of no-contact interventions with college students. First, the interventions vary widely in length, ranging from four 20-minute sessions (47) to one 1-minute session (46). Second, the interventions varied in the type of information provided to students, with effective interventions using different combinations of skills-based information, personalized normative feedback, alcohol consequences, physiological information on BAC, tolerance, and metabolism, feedback on money spent and calories consumed, advice on responsible drinking, and information on resources on how to change drinking. Determining the necessary components is important in maintaining brevity of assessment and information while still ensuring an adequate dose of intervention. The studies also have different results on which drinking variables are affected by the intervention, whether it reduces overall quantity, heaviest drinking day, alcohol-related consequences, or peak BAC. There does not seem to be a general pattern in which outcome variables are most affected by no-contact interventions. Examination of the components to the interventions that may target specific drinking patterns may help to better increase their overall benefits.

Determining how these no-contact interventions lead to decreases in drinking is another area for future research. Two studies attempted to demonstrate that changes in perceived discrepancy mediate the interventions' effect on drinking behavior. Neighbors and colleagues (46) found that the intervention group had greater reductions in perceived drinking norms, which was a mediator of the effects of the PNF on drinking behaviors, and while Collins et al. (38) found that the intervention groups had higher perceived discrepancies between their and their peers' drinking, discrepancy was not a mediator of the intervention's effect on drinking. Further investigation of the relative impact of changes in perceived norms, discrepancies, and motivation to change would help identify the most important elements in these interventions.

While the no-contact interventions are of comparable efficacy to in-person interventions in the short-term, the effects may disappear in longer-term follow-up. Future research may focus on ways to either amplify the effects of the intervention or lengthen treatment effects. Research that has used repeated mailings (37) may lengthen treatment effects, and future studies may more systematically investigate the effect of additional reminder or booster-session e-mails or mailings on the potential for a longer-term impact of the intervention. Including reminder e-mails, mailings, exercises, or progress reports may help extend effects of the intervention.

Finally, future research with other forms of mailed interventions or technologies such as cellular phones (61) or instant messaging could broaden the modalities available for no-contact interventions. For example, another no-contact intervention to explore is interactive voice response (IVR) technology. IVR uses computer-based telephone systems to make and receive calls, and provide and collect information. IVR has been successfully used for purposes of assessment, screening, monitoring, and assisting with health behavior change (62,63), has been found to reduce relapse to pain behavior following Cognitive Behavioral Therapy for chronic pain (64), and has shown promise as a supplement to a brief motivational interview for HIV patients (65). IVR could be examined for use in the college student population to provide personalized and normative feedback, provide educational information, and monitor drinking behavior over time.

While there are gaps in our knowledge on the effectiveness of no-contact interventions with college students, current evidence from studies that have included a comparison group with interventionist contact suggests that brief interventions that do not require therapist contact show similar efficacy to those interventions that do. Especially with internet-based interventions, no-contact interventions provide a less costly and perhaps effective way to reach a larger number of people than in-person interventions can, and provide interactive and personalized interventions in a way that mass-media campaigns cannot. Providing students with risk assessments and normative information before or shortly after they begin school may prove to be a powerful preventative measure in reducing the negative effects of alcohol use on the college population.

REFERENCES

1. Saitz R: Unhealthy alcohol use. N Engl J Med 2005; 352: 596-607. doi: 10.1056/NEJMcp042262
2. Hingson RW, Heeren T, Zakocs RC, Kopstein A, Wechsler H: Magnitude of alcohol-related mortality and morbidity among U.S. college students ages 18-24. J Stud Alcohol 2002; 63: 136-144.
3. Wechsler H, Lee JE, Kuo M, Lee H: College binge drinking in the 1990s: A continuing problem. Results of the Harvard School of Public Health 1999 College Alcohol Study. J Am Coll Health 2000; 48: 199-210.
4. Wechsler H, Lee JE, Kuo M, Seibring M, Nelson TF, Lee H: Trends in college binge drinking during a period of increased prevention efforts. J Am Coll Health 2002; 50: 203-217.
5. Knight JR, Wechsler H, Kuo M, Seibring M, Weitzman ER, Schuckit MA: Alcohol abuse and dependence among U.S. college students. J Stud Alcohol 2002; 63: 263-270.
6. Larimer ME, Cronce JM: Identification, prevention, and treatment: A review of individual-focused strategies to reduce problematic alcohol consumption by college students. J Stud Alcohol 2002; 14(suppl): 148-163.
7. Darkes J, Goldman MS: Expectancy challenge and drinking reduction: Experimental evidence for a mediational process. J Consult Clin Psychol 1993; 61: 344-353.
8. Darkes J, Goldman MS: Expectancy challenge and drinking reduction: Process and structure in the alcohol expectancy network. Exp Clin Psychopharmacol 1998; 6: 64-76. doi: 10.1037/1064-1297.6.1.64
9. Cronin C: Harm reduction for alcohol-use-related problems among college students. Subst Use Misuse 1996; 31: 2029-2037.
10. Garvin RB, Alcorn JD, Faulkner KK: Behavioral strategies for alcohol abuse prevention with high-risk college males. Journal of Alcohol and Drug Education 1990; 36: 23-34.
11. Baer JS, Marlatt GA, Kivlahan DR, Fromme K: An experimental test of three methods of alcohol risk reduction with young adults. J Consult Clin Psychol 1992; 60: 974-979. doi: 10.1037/0022-006X.60.6.974
12. Kivlahan DR, Marlatt GA, Fromme K, Coppel DB, Williams E: Secondary prevention with college drinkers: Evaluation of an alcohol skills training program. J Consult Clin Psychol 1990; 58: 805-810. doi: 10.1037/0022-006X.58.6.805
13. Borsari B, Carey KB: Effects of a brief motivational intervention with college student drinkers. J Consult Clin Psychol 2000; 68: 728-733. doi: 10.1037/0022-006X.68.4.728
14. Larimer ME, Turner AP, Anderson BK, Fader JS, Kilmer JR, Palmer RS, Cronce JM: Evaluating a brief alcohol intervention with fraternities. J Stud Alcohol 2001; 62: 370-380.

15. Marlatt GA, Baer JS, Kivlahan DR, Dimeff LA, Larimer ME, Quigley LA, Somers JM, Williams E: Screening and brief intervention for high-risk college student drinkers: Results from a two-year follow-up assessment. J Consult Clin Psychol 1998; 66: 604-615. doi: 10.1037/0022-006X.66.4.604

16. Greenfield SF, Keliher A, Sugarman D: Who comes to voluntary, community-based alcohol screening? Results of the First Annual National Alcohol Screening Day, 1999. Am J Psychiatry 2003; 160: 1677-1683. doi: 10.1176/appi.ajp.160.9.1677

17. Black DR, Coster DC: Interest in a stepped approach model (SAM): Identification of recruitment strategies for university alcohol programs. Health Education Quarterly 1996; 23: 98-114.

18. Foote J, Wilkens C, Vavagiakis P: A national survey of alcohol screening and referral in college health centers. J Am Coll Health 2004; 52: 149-157.

19. US Department of Commerce: A Nation Online: How Americans Are Expanding Their Use of the Internet. Washington, DC: US Dept of Commerce, Economics and Statistics Administration, National Telecommunications and Information Administration; February 2002.

20. Harris Interactive: College kids are the most wired group in the US. Available at: http://www.nua.ie/surveys/index.cgi?f = VS&art_id = 905358225&rel = true. Accessed July 5, 2005.

21. Jordan CM, Oei TPS: Help-seeking behaviour in problem drinkers: A review. British Journal of Addiction 1989; 84: 979-988.

22. Walters ST: In praise of feedback: An effective intervention for college students who are heavy drinkers. J Am Coll Health 2000; 48: 235-238.

23. Wing RR: Cross-cutting themes in maintenance of behavior change. Health Psychol 2000; 19: 84-88. doi: 10.1037/0278-6133.19.Suppl1.84

24. Humphreys K, Tucker JA: Toward more responsive and effective intervention systems for alcohol-related problems. Addiction 2002; 97: 126-132. doi: 10.1046/j.1360-0443.2002.00004.x

25. Hall MJ, Tidwell WC: Internet recovery for substance abuse and alcoholism: An exploratory study of services users. J Subst Abuse Treat 2003; 24: 161-167. doi: 10.1016/S0740-5472(02)00355-0

26. Cloud RN, Peacock PL: Internet screening and interventions for problem drinking: Results from the www.carebetter.com pilot study. Alcoholism Treatment Quarterly 2001; 19: 23-44. doi: 10.1300/J020v19n02_02

27. Cunningham JA, Humphreys K, Koski-Jannes A: Providing personalized assessment feedback for problem drinkers on the Internet: A pilot project. J Stud Alcohol 2000; 61: 794-798.

28. Saitz R, Helmuth ED, Aromaa SE, Guard A, Belanger M, Rosenbloom DL: Web-based screening and brief intervention for the spectrum of alcohol problems. Prev Med 2004; 39: 969-975. doi: 10.1016/j.ypmed.2004.04.011

29. Koski-Jannes A, Cunningham J: Interest in different forms of self-help in a general population of drinkers. Addict Behav 2001; 26: 91-99. doi: 10.1016/S0306-4603(00)00092-7

30. Kypri K, Saunders JB, Gallagher SJ: Acceptability of various brief intervention approaches for hazardous drinking among university students. Alcohol Alcohol 2003; 38: 626-628. doi: 10.1093/alcalc/agg121

31. Walters ST, Miller E, Chiauzzi E: Wired for wellness: E-interventions for addressing college drinking. J Subst Abuse Treat 2005; 29: 139-145. doi: 10.1016/j.jsat.2005.05.006

32. Murphy JG, Benson TA, Vuchinich RE, Deskins MM, Eakin D, Flood AM, McDevitt-Murphy ME, Torrealday O: A comparison of personalized feedback for college student drinkers delivered with and without a motivational interview. J Stud Alcohol 2004; 65: 200-203.

33. Sharmer L: Evaluation of alcohol education programs on attitude, knowledge, and self-reported behavior of college students. Evaluation & the Health Professions 2001; 24: 336-357. doi: 10.1177/01632780122034957

34. White HR, Morgan TJ, Pugh LA, Celinska K, Labouvie EW, Pandina RJ: Evaluating two brief substance-use interventions for mandated college students. J Stud Alcohol 2006; 67: 309-317.

35. Agostinelli G, Brown JM, Miller WR: Effects of normative feedback on consumption among heavy drinking colleges students. J Drug Educ 1995; 25: 31-40.

36. Miller WR, Sovereign RG, Krege B: Motivational interviewing with problem drinkers II: The Drinker's Check-up as a preventive intervention. Behavioural Psychotherapy 1988; 16: 251-268.

37. Saunders JB, Kypros K, Walters ST, Laforge RG, Larimer ME: Approaches to brief intervention for hazardous drinking in young people. Alcohol Clin Exp Res 2004; 28: 322-329. doi: 10.1097/01.ALC.0000113418.12889.08

38. Collins SE, Carey KB, Sliwinski MJ: Mailed personalized normative feedback as a brief intervention for at-risk college drinkers. J Stud Alcohol 2002; 63: 559-567.

39. Walters ST, Bennett ME, Miller JE: Reducing alcohol use in college students: A controlled trial of two brief interventions. J Drug Educ 2000; 30: 361-372. doi: 10.2190/JHML-0JPD-YE7L-14CT

40. Johnsson KO, Berglund M: Comparison between a cognitive behavioural alcohol programme and post-mailed minimal intervention in high-risk drinking university freshmen: results from a randomized controlled trial. Alcohol Alcohol 2006; 41: 174-180. doi: 10.1093/alcalc/agh243

41. Saunders JB, Aasland OG, Babor TF: Development of the Alcohol Use Disorders Identification Test (AUDIT): WHO collaborative project on early detection of persons with harmful alcohol consumption: II. Addiction, 1993; 88: 791-804.

42. Dimeff LA, Baer JS, Kivlahan DR, Marlatt GA: Brief Alcohol Screening and Intervention for College Students. New York, NY: Guilford Press; 1999.

43. Hester RK, Delaney HD: Behavioral Self-Control Program for Windows: Results of a controlled clinical trial. J Consult Clin Psychol 1997; 65: 686-693. doi: 10.1037/0022-006X.65.4.686

44. Hester RK, Squires DD, Delaney HD: The Drinker's Check-up: 12-month outcomes of a controlled clinical trial of a stand-alone software program for problem drinkers. J Subst Abuse Treat 2005; 28: 159-169. doi: 10.1016/j.jsat.2004.12.002

45. Kypri K, Saunders JB, Williams SM, McGee RO, Langley JD, Cashell-Smith ML, Gallagher SJ: Web-based screening and brief intervention for hazardous drinking: A double-blind randomized controlled trial. Addiction 2004; 99: 1410-1417. doi: 10.1111/j.1360-0443.2004.00847.x

46. Neighbors C, Larimer ME, Lewis MA: Targeting misperceptions of descriptive drinking norms: Efficacy of a computer-delivered personalized normative feedback intervention. J Consult Clin Psychol 2004; 72: 434-447. doi: 10.1037/0022-006X.72.3.434

47. Chiauzzi E, Green TC, Lord S, Thum C, Goldstein M: My Student Body: A high-risk drinking prevention web site for college students. J Am Coll Health 2005; 53: 263-274.

48. Moore MJ, Soderquist J, Werch C: Feasibility and efficacy of a binge drinking prevention intervention for college students delivered via the internet versus postal mail. J Am Coll Health 2005; 54: 38-44.

49. Witte K, Meyer G, Martell D: Effective Health Risk Messages: A Step-By-Step Guide. Thousand Oaks, CA: Sage Publications, 2001.

50. Saitz R, Palfai TP, Freedner N, Winter MR, Macdonald A, Lu J, Ozonoff A, Rosenbloom D, Dejong W: Screening and brief intervention online for college students: the iHealth study. Alcohol Alcohol 2007; 42: 28-36. doi: 10.1093/alcalc/agl092.

51. Kypri K: Electronic screening and brief intervention (e-SBI) for hazardous drinking: a four-arm randomized controlled trial. Alcohol Clin Exp Res. 2005; 29: 73A.

52. Miller ET: Preventing alcohol abuse and alcohol-related negative consequences among freshmen college students: Using emerging computer technology to deliver and evaluate the effectiveness of brief intervention efforts. Dissertation Abstracts International: Section B: The Sciences & Engineering 2001; 61(8-B): 4417.

53. Steiner JW, Woodall WG, Yeagley JA: The E-Chug: A randomized, controlled study of a web-based binge drinking intervention with college freshman. Poster Presented at: Society for Prevention Research; May 2005; Washington, DC.

54. Walters ST, Hester RK, Chiauzzi E, Miller E: Demon rum: High-tech solutions to an age-old problem. Alcohol Clin Exp Res. 2005; 29: 270-277. doi: 10.1097/01.ALC.0000153543.03339.81

55. Hester RK: Behavioral self-control training. In: Hester RK, Miller WR, eds. Handbook of Alcoholism Treatment Approaches: Effective Alternatives. Needham Heights, MA: Allyn & Bacon; 1995: 148-159.

56. Moyer A, Finney JW, Swearingen CE, Vergun P: Brief interventions for alcohol problems: A meta-analytic review of controlled investigations in treatment-seeking and non-treatment-seeking populations. Addiction 2002; 97: 279-292. doi: 10.1046/j.1360-0443.2002.00018.x

57. Cunningham JA, Wild TC, Bondy SJ, Lin E: Impact of normative feedback on problem drinkers: A small-area population study. J Stud Alcohol 2001; 62: 228-233.

58. Walters ST, Woodall WG: Mailed feedback reduces consumption among moderate drinkers who are employed. Prevention Science 2003; 4: 287-294. doi: 10.1023/A:1026024400450

59. Posavac EJ: College students' views of excessive drinking and the university's role. J Drug Educ 1993; 23: 237-245.

60. Stewart SH, Conrod PJ, Marlatt GA, Comeau N, Thush C, Krank M: New developments in prevention and early intervention for alcohol abuse in youths. Alcohol Clin Exp Res 2005; 29: 278-286. doi: 10.1097/01.ALC.0000153547.34399.E8

61. Obermayer JL, Riley WT, Asif O: College smoking-cessation using cell phone text messaging. J Am Coll Health 2004; 53: 71-78.

62. Corkrey R, Parkinson L: Interactive voice response: Review of studies 1989-2000. Behavior Research Methods, Instruments & Computers 2002; 34: 342-353.

63. Glasgow RE, Bull SS, Piette JD: Interactive behavior change technology: A partial solution to the competing demands of primary care. Am J Prev Med 2004; 27: 80-87. doi: 10.1016/j.amepre.2004.04.026

64. Naylor MR, Helzer JE, Naud S: Automated telephone as an adjunct for the treatment of chronic pain: A pilot study. Journal of Pain 2002; 3: 429-438. doi: 10.1054/jpai.2002.129563

65. Aharonovich E, Hatzenbuehler M, Yao P, Johnson B, O'Leary A, Hasin D: A low-cost, sustainable intervention for drinking reduction in the HIV primary care setting. Presented at: Twenty-Eighth Annual Meeting of the Research Society on Alcoholism; 2005; Santa Barbara, CA.

doi:10.1300/J465v28n04_04

Measuring Performance of Brief Alcohol Counseling in Medical Settings: A Review of the Options and Lessons from the Veterans Affairs (VA) Health Care System

Katharine A. Bradley, MD, MPH
Emily C. Williams, MPH
Carol E. Achtmeyer, MN
Eric J. Hawkins, PhD
Alex H. S. Harris, PhD, MS
Madeleine S. Frey, BA
Thomas Craig, MD, MPH
Daniel R. Kivlahan, PhD

Katharine A. Bradley is affiliated with Health Services Research & Development, Primary and Specialty Medical Care, Center of Excellence in Substance Abuse Treatment and Education, VA Puget Sound Health Care System, Seattle, WA, and the Departments of Medicine and Health Services, University of Washington, Seattle, WA.

Emily C. Williams is affiliated with Health Services Research & Development and Center of Excellence in Substance Abuse Treatment and Education, VA Puget Sound Health Care System, Seattle, WA, and the Departments of Medicine and Health Services as well as the Graduate School of Public Health and Community Medicine, University of Washington, Seattle, WA.

Carol E. Achtmeyer is affiliated with Health Services Research & Development, Primary and Specialty Medical Care, and Center of Excellence in Substance Abuse Treatment and Education, VA Puget Sound Health Care System, Seattle, WA.

Eric J. Hawkins is affiliated with Health Services Research & Development, Center of Excellence in Substance Abuse Treatment and Education, VA Puget Sound Health Care System, Seattle, WA, and the Department of Psychiatry and Behavioral Sciences, University of Washington, Seattle, WA.

Alex H. S. Harris is affiliated with the Center for Health Care Evaluation, VA Palo Alto Health Care System, Menlo Park, CA.

Madeleine S. Frey is affiliated with Health Services Research & Development, VA Puget Sound Health Care System, Seattle, WA, and the Department of Health Services, University of Washington, Seattle, WA.

Thomas Craig is affiliated with the Office of Quality and Performance, Veterans Health Administration, Washington, DC.

Daniel R. Kivlahan is affiliated with Health Services Research & Development, Center of Excellence in Substance Abuse Treatment and Education, VA Puget Sound Health Care System, Seattle, WA, and the Department of Psychiatry and Behavioral Sciences, University of Washington, Seattle, WA.

Address correspondence to: Katharine A. Bradley, MD, MPH, HSR&D (152), VA Puget Sound Health Services Research & Development, 1100 Olive Way, Suite 1400, Seattle, WA 98101 (E-mail: willi@u.washington.edu).

The research reported here was supported by the Department of Veterans Affairs, Veterans Health Administration, Health Services Research and Development Service. The manuscript was specifically produced with support from the Veterans Affairs Substance Use Disorders Quality Enhancement Research Initiative (SUD QUERI; SUB 98-000) and Center of Excellence in Substance Abuse Treatment & Education. Drs. Kivlahan and Bradley presently serve as the Clinical Coordinator and Co-Clinical Coordinator of the SUD QUERI.

The authors would like to acknowledge Roxane Rusch, RN and Bryan Volpp, MD for their collaboration and for assisting us in obtaining and interpreting quality improvement data presented in this report.

The views expressed in this article are those of the authors and do not necessarily reflect the position or policy of the Department of Veterans Affairs or the University of Washington.

[Haworth co-indexing entry note]: "Measuring Performance of Brief Alcohol Counseling in Medical Settings: A Review of the Options and Lessons from the Veterans Affairs (VA) Health Care System." Bradley, Katharine A. et al. Co-published simultaneously in *Substance Abuse* (The Haworth Medical Press, an imprint of The Haworth Press, Inc.) Vol. 28, No. 4, 2007, pp. 133-149; and: *Alcohol/Drug Screening and Brief Intervention: Advances in Evidence-Based Practice* (ed: Richard Saitz, and Marc Galanter) The Haworth Medical Press, an imprint of The Haworth Press, Inc., 2007, pp. 133-149. Single or multiple copies of this article are available for a fee from The Haworth Document Delivery Service [1-800-HAWORTH, 9:00 a.m. - 5:00 p.m. (EST). E-mail address: docdelivery@haworthpress.com].

Available online at http://suba.haworthpress.com
doi:10.1300/J465v28n04_05

SUMMARY. Brief alcohol counseling is a top US prevention priority but has not been widely implemented. The lack of an easy performance measure for brief alcohol counseling is one important barrier to implementation. The purpose of this report is to outline important issues related to measuring performance of brief alcohol counseling in health care settings. We review the strengths and limitations of several options for measuring performance of brief alcohol counseling and describe three measures of brief alcohol counseling tested in the Veterans Affairs (VA) Health Care System. We conclude that administrative data are not well-suited to measuring performance of brief alcohol counseling. Patient surveys appear to offer the optimal approach currently available for comparing performance of brief alcohol counseling *across* health care systems, while more options are available for measuring performance *within* health care systems. Further research is needed in this important area of quality improvement. doi:10.1300/J465v28n04_05 *[Article copies available for a fee from The Haworth Document Delivery Service: 1-800-HAWORTH. E-mail address: <docdelivery@haworthpress.com> Website: <http://www.HaworthPress.com>]*

KEYWORDS. Quality improvement, performance measurement, alcohol screening, brief intervention, brief alcohol counseling, implementation, primary care

INTRODUCTION

Brief alcohol counseling for patients who drink excessively is widely recommended (1, 2) and has been designated one of the top 10 prevention priorities for the US (3). A US study showed that for every dollar spent on alcohol screening and brief alcohol counseling, costs to the health care system decreased by $4.30 over the following 4 years (4-6). However, implementation of brief alcohol counseling has lagged behind other important preventive health priorities (7, 8). The lack of a well-defined, efficient method for measuring performance of brief alcohol counseling has likely contributed to slow implementation (9, 10).

Improving the quality of health care requires being able to define, operationalize, and measure quality (10-12). Within health care organizations, systematic measurement of care is used to identify gaps in quality, design systems to improve care, and subsequently evaluate whether quality improvement efforts have been successful. Standardized performance measurement also permits comparison across health care systems (13, 14).

Although there has been increasing interest in developing standardized measures to improve the quality of mental health care (15, 16), and performance measures for substance use disorder treatment are being developed by national organizations (e.g., National Quality Forum, the Washington Circle, Substance Abuse and Mental Health Services Administration, and the National Committee for Quality Assurance), there is no consensus or recommendation for measuring performance of brief alcohol counseling. A performance measure of brief alcohol counseling would allow health care organizations to determine whether evidence-based alcohol counseling was being offered to appropriate patients and facilitate the evaluation of quality improvement efforts to address identified deficits. Such a measure would also permit comparisons of brief alcohol counseling performance across health care organizations.

However, measuring the performance of brief alcohol counseling is challenging. Health care performance measures must specify which patients should receive a certain aspect of evidence-based care and provide criteria for determining which patients have received the desired care. These are the denominator and the numerator of a performance measure, respectively. Further, performance measures designed to compare health care systems must rely on standardized, commonly available data. Currently, no measures are in widespread use that identify patients with alcohol misuse, the target population for brief alcohol counseling, or indicate when brief alcohol counseling has occurred.

The purpose of this report is to outline the strengths and limitations of commonly considered approaches to performance measurement of brief alcohol counseling. We address performance measures for evaluating brief alcohol counseling within health care organizations as well as for comparing brief alcohol counseling across health care systems. First, we discuss the appropriate target population for brief alcohol counseling–the denominator of a performance measure. Second, we address the definition and measurement of brief alcohol counseling– the numerator of a performance measure. Third, we consider the strengths and limitations of four types of data for measuring performance of brief alcohol counseling: administrative data; patient surveys; manual medical record reviews; and data from clinical decision support software in electronic medical records (EMRs). Finally, we review the Veterans Affairs (VA) Health Care System's experience pilot-testing several approaches to measuring brief alcohol counseling performance. Although there are limitations to what any performance measure can achieve, we conclude that certain approaches to measuring performance will be more likely than others to promote implementation of evidence-based brief alcohol counseling.

THE DENOMINATOR OF A PERFORMANCE MEASURE FOR BRIEF ALCOHOL COUNSELING

Who Should Receive Brief Alcohol Counseling? Patients with alcohol misuse constitute the target population for brief alcohol counseling. Alcohol misuse includes a spectrum from risky drinking to alcohol use disorders (9, 17). Although many patients with milder alcohol misuse will not progress to more severe problem drinking, they are nonetheless at increased risk for trauma (18) and other adverse medical outcomes (19). Moreover, these patients with milder, nondependent alcohol misuse might be the most likely to respond to brief alcohol counseling (17, 20-22).

Although some meta-analyses supporting the efficacy of brief alcohol counseling have concluded that patients with alcohol dependence may not respond (20), there are several reasons these patients should be included in the denominator for a performance measure of brief alcohol counseling. First, research on alcohol dependent patients in treatment suggests that recollection of alcohol-related advice from a physician is associated with improved outcomes (23), and brief alcohol counseling could increase patient acceptance of referral or catalyze changes in drinking even in those who do not follow-through with referral (24, 25). Second, reliably identifying alcohol dependent patients would require in-depth diagnostic interviews that are not feasible in many clinical settings. Finally, and most importantly, several recent effectiveness trials have not excluded alcohol dependent patients (26-28), and have found a beneficial effect of brief alcohol counseling (26-28). For these reasons, alcohol dependent patients should not be excluded from the denominator of a performance measure for brief alcohol counseling.

Should Clinician Identification of Alcohol Misuse Be Used to Define the Target Population? Many performance measures rely on diagnoses documented by providers to identify the target population–the denominator of a performance measure. However, alcohol misuse is not a diagnosis per se, and therefore there is no ICD-9 code for alcohol misuse. Further, relying on clinician documentation to identify patients who misuse alcohol would have two important limitations (Table 1). First, up to two-thirds of patients with alcohol misuse would not be identified by providers because clinicians usually do not recognize alcohol misuse in the absence of systematic alcohol screening (29-33).

Second, relying on providers to identify patients with alcohol misuse would bias performance measurement of brief alcohol counseling. Even when providers do identify patients with alcohol misuse, they are most likely to recognize and counsel patients with the most severe alcohol-related problems (29, 31, 34, 35). In one observational study, rates of brief alcohol counseling reported by patients who screened positive for alcohol misuse ranged from 13% among patients with the mildest alcohol misuse to 71% among those with the most severe misuse (29). To understand how this could bias a performance measure of brief alcohol counseling, assume that we wanted to compare performance in two identical health care systems, each with a 24% prevalence of alcohol misuse (9). Assume further that one of these health care systems had an alcohol misuse screening program and the other did not. In the

TABLE 1. Major Limitations and Challenges Associated with Potential Measures of the Denominator and Numerator of a Brief Alcohol Counseling Performance Measure

DENOMINATOR	**LIMITATIONS AND CHALLENGES**
Patients with alcohol misuse identified by provider documentation	• Relies on provider recognition and documentation of alcohol misuse, limited due to evidence that providers: -- miss the majority of alcohol misuse -- identify only the most severe problem drinkers • Could bias performance measurement and could thereby discourage systematic alcohol screening
All outpatients	• Does not evaluate whether patients who misuse alcohol received brief alcohol counseling • Could be biased due to local variation in the prevalence of alcohol misuse and severe alcohol misuse • Does not encourage alcohol screening, which might be an essential component of brief alcohol counseling
Patients who screen positive for alcohol misuse	• Requires population-based alcohol misuse screening which is not routine in many outpatient settings • Requires standardization of alcohol screening instrument and threshold for the performance measure • Potentially biased by recall, social desirability, and non-response
NUMERATOR	
Nonspecific provider documentation of brief alcohol counseling	• Does not assess quality or content of brief alcohol counseling • In systems with electronic medical record, one mouse click could automatically document counseling, which might not reflect quality
Nonspecific patient report that they received brief alcohol counseling	• Does not assess quality or content of brief alcohol counseling • Potentially biased by recall, social desirability, and non-response
Provider documentation that alcohol-related advice & feedback were offered	• Requires a consensus on required components of brief alcohol counseling • Details of brief alcohol counseling provided may not always be documented • In systems with electronic medical records, one mouse click could automatically document counseling, which might not reflect quality
Patient reports that they were offered alcohol-related advice & feedback	• Requires a consensus on required components of brief alcohol counseling • Potentially biased by recall, social desirability, and non-response

system without screening, about 33% of the 24% of patients with alcohol misuse would typically be identified, or 8% of the entire population (33% × 24%), whereas in the system with screening, 100% of patients who screened positive for alcohol misuse would be identified, or 24% of the total population. Further, in the system without screening, a relatively high proportion of identified patients would be counseled–perhaps 60%–since predominantly patients with severe alcohol misuse would be identified. In contrast, in the system with screening, a lower proportion of identified patients would be counseled–perhaps 30%–since more patients with milder alcohol misuse would be included in the denominator (29). Paradoxically, in the first system without screening, a high proportion of identified patients would be counseled, but only 4.8% of the total patient population would be counseled (60% × 8%), whereas in the system with screening and a lower proportion of identified patients counseled, 7.2% of the total population would be counseled (30% × 24%). In other words, the system that only assessed whether brief alcohol counseling was offered to patients whose alcohol misuse was recognized by providers would appear to provide brief alcohol counseling to a higher proportion of patients (60% vs. 30%), when in fact a lower proportion of the total population was being counseled (4.8% vs. 7.2%). Therefore, relying on providers to identify patients with alcohol misuse for the denominator of a performance measure could create a disincentive for systems to appropriately implement routine alcohol screening.

Should Performance of Brief Alcohol Counseling Be Measured in All Outpatients? Since we cannot rely on providers to identify patients with alcohol misuse in the absence of routine screening, a possible alternative would be to assess brief alcohol counseling among all patients in a given health care system. This would greatly simplify performance measurement, but would have three important limitations (Table 1). First, evaluating the proportion of all outpatients who received brief alcohol counseling would not indicate whether patients with alcohol misuse were counseled. Health care systems might offer routine health promotion appointments counseling patients about appropriate alcohol use, but the participants in such a program would likely be the most health conscious patients who might not need brief alcohol counseling. Second, assessing brief alcohol counseling in a denominator of all outpatients would unfairly ignore variability in the prevalence of alcohol misuse across systems. Systems with a lower prevalence of alcohol misuse, perhaps due to a higher proportion of women or older patients, could appear to perform poorly even though they might be offering brief alcohol counseling to appropriate patients. While effects of demographic characteristics could be adjusted for statistically, adjustments for local variation in alcohol use and misuse would be difficult. Finally, assessment of drinking likely contributes to the efficacy of brief alcohol counseling (36, 37), and brief alcohol counseling has never been evaluated without prior alcohol screening. For these reasons, a system that measured the performance of brief alcohol counseling in all patients would not assess whether evidence-based brief alcohol screening and counseling had been implemented.

Use of Screening Questionnaires to Identify Alcohol Misuse. Because of the limitations of the above approaches, alcohol screening is necessary to identify the appropriate patients for the denominator of a performance measure of brief alcohol counseling. Since no valid laboratory test is yet widely available for alcohol misuse screening (38), patient report on validated alcohol screening questionnaires is currently the optimal approach. However, there are several challenges to using alcohol screening questionnaires to identify patients with alcohol misuse (Table 1). First, alcohol screening has not been widely implemented. Second, use of alcohol screening questionnaires for performance measurement would require consensus on a standard approach to alcohol screening including specifying an instrument and threshold to permit comparisons across health care systems. Such a consensus on a standard approach to alcohol screening does not currently exist. Third, although validated screening questionnaires offer the most effective approach to identifying alcohol misuse, they are susceptible to recall, social desirability and response biases.

Which Screening Questionnaires for Alcohol Misuse Are Valid and Feasible? There are two practical approaches to brief alcohol screening that could identify patients with alcohol misuse for the denominator of a performance measure. The first option is to use one of several effective single-item screening tests that ask about the recency or frequency of heavy drinking (≥ 5 drinks on an occasion for men and ≥ 4 drinks on an occasion for women) (39, 40). For example, the National Institute on Alcohol Abuse and Alcoholism recommends asking patients who drink alcohol: "How many times in the past year have you had 5 or more drinks in a day (4 or more for women)?" Another option is the 3-item AUDIT-C used to screen for alcohol misuse in the VA (41-45). Although longer, the AUDIT-C has the advantage of providing information about a patient's typical drinking pattern, severity of alcohol misuse (19, 46, 47), and readiness to change (48). Questionnaires designed to identify patients with alcohol use disorders (e.g., CAGE) should not be used because they are insensitive for identifying patients with risky drinking (9).

However, in order to make performance measures acceptable to clinicians and managers, the screening thresholds used in clinical practice may be too sensitive and therefore result in too many false positives for a performance measure. In clinical practice, patients found to have false positive screening tests can be briefly educated about recommended drinking limits (43), so screening thresholds are often used that balance sensitivity and specificity (41). When alcohol screening is used to define the denominator of a performance measure, however, false positive screening tests may have higher costs. If clinicians feel they are expected to offer unnecessary care (i.e., counsel patients who do not misuse alcohol), it could lead to questions about the appropriateness of the performance measure, thereby undermining the purpose of the measure (49). Given this potential added "cost" of false positive screening tests when used for performance measurement, a higher screening threshold may be justified. For the two approaches to screening above, reasonable options to identify the denominator of a performance measure of brief alcohol counseling are report of heavy drinking monthly or more often or an AUDIT-C score > 5 (43).

Should Alcohol Misuse and Drug Abuse Screening Be Combined? Some policymakers advocate combining alcohol and (non-nicotine) drug abuse screening to identify the denominator of a performance measure. However, there is currently no evidence or expert consensus to support the benefit of population-based screening and brief intervention for other substance use disorders. The proven benefits of brief alcohol counseling (3, 17, 20) combined with the burden of alcohol misuse, therefore distinguish alcohol screening from screening for other drug abuse (50), and routine outpatient screening for other drug abuse is not currently recommended (51).

THE NUMERATOR OF A PERFORMANCE MEASURE OF BRIEF ALCOHOL COUNSELING

What Is Brief Alcohol Counseling? In this section we discuss the definition of brief alcohol counseling before reviewing approaches for distinguishing patients who receive it (i.e., the numerator for a performance measure). Although telephone and web-based interventions for alcohol misuse have been developed and tested, most trials of brief alcohol counseling in medical settings have evaluated face to face counseling interventions (17, 20-22, 52-55), and this review focuses on performance measurement of brief alcohol counseling in outpatient medical settings.

There is substantial variation in the brief alcohol counseling interventions found to be efficacious in randomized controlled trials. At one extreme, some trials in medical settings studied relatively long motivational interviewing interventions conducted by mental health specialists (56). At the other extreme, five minute interventions by primary care clinicians providing brief advice and feedback on the health risks of drinking were shown to be as efficacious as longer counseling sessions (57). Other studies evaluated interventions delivered by primary care providers, based on concepts of motivational interviewing (24). These interventions typically combined advice and feedback with a menu of options, negotiation of a drinking goal, and other support such as workbooks (5, 27).

Of seven published reviews of brief alcohol counseling trials to date that have concluded that opportunistic brief alcohol counseling is efficacious (17, 20-22, 52-54), two have focused on outpatient settings and used standardized searches to identify trials (17, 21). In both reviews, advice and feedback linking alcohol use and health were the most common components of brief alcohol counseling noted. Feedback included either personalized feedback linking alcohol use to the patient's own health concerns or general feedback indicating that the patient was drinking at a level known to be unhealthy. All brief alcohol counseling trials have included alcohol screening, which might itself act as an intervention (37), and follow-up visits were also almost always included.

Non-Specific Measures of Brief Alcohol Counseling. One method for measuring brief alcohol counseling would be to rely on provider documentation or patient report that brief alcohol counseling was provided (yes/no). Non-specific measures are simplest to implement, as they can be obtained from medical records or billing sheets (provider documentation) or from mailed surveys (patient report). Furthermore, such non-specific measures of brief alcohol counseling do not require a consensus on the required components of brief alcohol counseling.

The Importance of Specific Measures of Brief Alcohol Counseling. An important limitation of relying on non-specific (yes/no) measures of performance is that they would not assess the quality of brief alcohol counseling. Audio-taped encounters suggest that primary care providers do not typically include advice and feedback in alcohol-related discussions with patients who misuse alcohol (58). In fact, clinicians appear uncomfortable or awkward, and instead change the subject or provide vague or ambiguous information (59). These and other data lead us to conclude that clinicians do not routinely offer patients evidence-based brief alcohol counseling even when alcohol-related discussions occur. Therefore, the quality of brief alcohol counseling is important, and a non-specific performance measure that only required providers or patients to indicate if alcohol-related counseling had occurred would not assess the quality of this important aspect of preventive care. For these reasons a performance measure that assesses specific dimension(s) of evidence-based brief alcohol counseling (e.g., advice and feedback) is needed.

In sum, the denominator of a performance measure of brief alcohol counseling should be based on a specified, validated brief screen for alcohol misuse (Table 1). The numerator of a performance measure for brief alcohol counseling needs to not only assess the proportion of patients who receive brief alcohol counseling, but also the quality of that counseling. In order to accomplish this, the numerator of a performance measure should evaluate whether providers offer patients with alcohol misuse both (1) explicit advice to drink within recommended limits or abstain and (2) feedback linking alcohol use to health.

APPROACHES TO MEASURING PERFORMANCE OF BRIEF ALCOHOL COUNSELING

The ideal performance measure for brief alcohol counseling would provide accurate measurement of the denominator (i.e., "Which patients are eligible for brief alcohol counseling due to alcohol misuse?") and the numerator (i.e., "Did eligible patients receive advice and feedback about the association of alcohol use and health?"), with readily available, reliable data, at an affordable cost. To our knowledge, strategies that have been discussed or tested as possible approaches to measuring performance of brief alcohol counseling rely on one of four types of data: administrative data, patient surveys, data abstracted by manual medical record review, or electronic data from clinical activity documented with clinical decision support software. While each approach has limitations for measuring the performance of brief alcohol counseling (Table 2), some approaches offer important advantages over others for promoting high quality, evidence-based brief alcohol counseling.

Administrative Data. Many performance measures use diagnostic, visit, billing, or procedure codes available in administrative data. For example, the National Committee for Quality Assurance (NCQA) Health Plan Employer Data and Information Set (HEDIS) performance measure for the "initiation and engagement of alcohol or drug dependence treatment"

TABLE 2. Four Types of Data for Measuring Brief Alcohol Counseling Performance: Limitations Related to Feasibility

	Administrative Data	**Patient Surveys**	**Manual Medical Record Review**	**Electronic Monitoring w/ Computerized Clinical Support**
Cannot currently identify patients with alcohol misuse (denominator)	X			
Cannot currently identify specific components of brief alcohol counseling	X			
Cannot currently distinguish alcohol and other drug counseling	X			
Cannot prompt providers to screen and offer brief alcohol counseling	X	X	X	
Potentially biased denominator due to low response		X		
Potentially biased denominator due to low screening rates			X	X
Large upfront investment in infrastructure			X	X
High ongoing measurement costs			X	
Cannot currently compare across health care systems in US				X
Extended time lag in data availability		X		
Limited to health care systems with electronic medical records				X

relies on International Classification of Disease (ICD) codes, Diagnosis Related Groups (DRGs), and Current Procedural Terminology (CPT) codes to evaluate treatment involvement (60-62).

Several types of administrative data have been considered potentially useful for measuring brief alcohol counseling performance. The Centers for Medicare and Medicaid Services (CMS) recently added two new billing codes to the Healthcare Common Procedure Coding System (HCPCS) that went into effect in January 2007: H0049 for alcohol/drug screening and H0050 for 15 minutes of alcohol/drug brief interventions (63). In addition, ICD-9 "V-codes," which are used when health care is not related to disease or injury, include a code for "counseling on substance use and abuse" (V65.42), which could be used to identify performance of brief alcohol counseling. Use of these administrative data for performance measurement could have significant advantages. Because these data are used for reimbursement they are readily available nationwide. This standardizes measurement and simplifies data collection across health care systems, markedly decreasing the cost of performance measurement.

However, administrative data also have important disadvantages for this type of performance measure. As noted above, there is currently no diagnostic code or other widely available administrative measure for the entire spectrum of alcohol misuse (the denominator). Since only 5-10% of primary care patients meet diagnostic criteria for alcohol use disorders, using existing ICD codes for alcohol use disorders would miss up to 20% of primary care patients who typically screen positive for the broader spectrum of alcohol misuse (64). The new HCPCS code (H0049) for alcohol/drug screening does not identify which patients screen positive. Further, even if a new ICD code for alcohol misuse were developed, relying on providers to identify alcohol misuse in the absence of standardized alcohol screening would miss the majority of patients who could benefit from brief alcohol counseling and would bias performance measurement. Administrative data also cannot currently identify the numerator for a performance measure of brief alcohol counseling. Neither H- nor V-codes (H0050 and V65.42) distinguish brief alcohol counseling from counseling for other drug abuse. Furthermore, non-specific procedure codes indicating brief alcohol counseling would provide no information on the quality of counseling.

Patient Surveys. Another approach to performance measurement of brief alcohol counseling would be to use patient surveys. For example, the Consumer Assessment of Healthcare Providers and Systems (CAHPS®), developed by the Agency for Healthcare Research and Quality (AHRQ), is used by NCQA to assess preventive care in addition to satisfaction, as part of its HEDIS performance measurement system. The 2007 CAHPS survey assesses whether patients received medical assistance with smoking cessation (65), but to date CAHPS has not been used to evaluate alcohol misuse or brief alcohol counseling.

Patient surveys have several strengths for performance measurement of brief alcohol counseling. First, a brief alcohol screening questionnaire can be embedded in surveys to identify patients with alcohol misuse, thus standardizing screening for performance measurement while allowing clinical practices the flexibility to choose their own screening protocols. In addition, using surveys to measure the performance of brief alcohol counseling emphasizes the patient perspective. This might encourage providers to focus on the brief alcohol counseling interaction rather than on non-specific documentation of alcohol counseling as an end in itself. Patient surveys could also capture specific components of brief alcohol counseling. A study that compared provider documentation to patient report found that rates of counseling based on patient report were generally higher than rates based on medical record documentation (66). Patient surveys can also be used to evaluate the quality of documented brief alcohol counseling, as has been done for alcohol screening (67).

However, patient surveys have several important limitations for measuring brief alcohol counseling performance. First, survey measures of brief alcohol counseling could be limited by response, recall, or social desirability biases. Conducting mailed patient surveys is also much more expensive than using administrative data for performance measurement and somewhat inefficient in that questions about alcohol would be mailed to all patients, even those who do not drink. Finally, the lag time between surveys and availability of data on performance is a disadvantage for quality improvement.

Manual Medical Record Review. Medical record reviews are commonly used for performance measurement. For example, health plans often report on HEDIS performance measures based on medical record reviews, and the VA has used medical record reviews extensively for quality improvement over the past decade (68). For brief alcohol counseling, medical record review can be used to evaluate the proportion of patients offered alcohol screening, identify patients with positive screens, and evaluate whether specific components of brief alcohol counseling are documented. Medical record review is attractive for performance measurement because it is flexible but standardized and can include care delivered over a specified time period (e.g., prior year). Medical record review can also obtain other important information (e.g., prior diagnoses of alcohol dependence) and can restrict assessment of brief alcohol counseling to eligible patients who screen positive for alcohol misuse.

Medical record review has several important limitations for measuring performance of brief alcohol counseling. First, behavioral counseling is often not documented in the medical record (66, 69). On the other hand, in settings with electronic medical records (EMRs) and clinical decision support, brief alcohol counseling could be documented so easily (e.g., with a single mouse click) that a broad array of counseling behavior could be reflected by uniform medical record documentation. This could make it difficult to assess the actual quality of brief alcohol counseling. In addition, for comparisons across health care systems, use of medical record review would require that all clinical alcohol screening be conducted with a uniform questionnaire and threshold. Finally, manual medical record review by trained abstractors is costly and requires large investments in infrastructure.

Clinical Decision Support Software That Prompts and Monitors Brief Alcohol Counseling. Large health care systems with EMRs routinely use clinical decision support software to prompt clinicians to provide desired care for specific patients while electronically monitoring documented care (70, 71). Clinical decision support systems could routinely prompt providers both to screen for alcohol misuse and offer brief alcohol counseling to appropriate patients. Such systems could also serve an educational function by requiring that providers document specific required components of brief alcohol counseling: alcohol-related advice and feedback (9). Further, these systems could monitor performance at relatively low cost.

However, EMRs require large up-front investments, and the design, programming and pilot testing of clinical decision support systems for brief alcohol counseling require a further commitment of clinician time and resources. In addition, little is known about the relationship between documentation of counseling by clicking boxes in an EMR and the quality of actual counseling provided. It may be too easy to document appropriate brief alcohol counseling. In other words, the quality of brief alcohol counseling provided may be limited due to lack of time or inadequate provider skill despite well documented brief alcohol counseling (59, 72). Moreover, EMRs differ across health care organizations and are not currently used by most US health care providers (73). Therefore, such systems are primarily useful for brief alcohol counseling quality improvement within a minority of health care systems and currently could not be used to compare care across all US health care systems.

PILOT TESTING MEASURES OF BRIEF ALCOHOL COUNSELING PERFORMANCE IN THE VA

The VA has made a major commitment to nationwide implementation of systematic alcohol misuse screening and development and testing of measures of brief alcohol counseling performance. In 2004, the VA Office of Quality and Performance (OQP) implemented screening for alcohol misuse as the first step towards implementation of brief alcohol counseling (9). Since that time, three approaches have been used to monitor performance of brief alcohol counseling among patients with alcohol misuse, permitting evaluation of the strengths and limitations of each approach. Below we present pilot data on these three approaches. This study was approved by the University of Washington Human Subjects Division and the VA Northern California Human Subjects Office, and a Data Use Agreement was obtained from the VA Office of Quality and Performance for these analyses.

Patient Surveys to Assess Alcohol-Related Advice. In 2004, the VA Survey of Healthcare Experiences of Patients (SHEP) was mailed monthly to randomly-selected outpatients who have had a recent appointment to assess patient satisfaction and other aspects of care. In 2004, when the VA began requiring that all outpatients be screened for alcohol misuse, the VA OQP began assessing alcohol misuse and brief alcohol counseling with SHEP. SHEP included the three AUDIT-C questions to screen for alcohol misuse and one question about alcohol-related advice: "In the past 12 months has a VA doctor or other VA health care provider advised you about your drinking (to drink less or not to drink alcohol)?" (9).

SHEP data from 2004 (Figure 1) showed that the proportion of patients who reported alcohol-related advice increased as the severity of alcohol misuse increased (9), consistent with previous research (29). These data also show that despite a higher proportion of patients with severe alcohol misuse reporting brief alcohol counseling than patients with mild/moderate alcohol misuse, the absolute number of patients with mild/moderate misuse who were counseled was greater since many more patients have mild-moderate misuse than have severe alcohol misuse. Moreover, the majority of patients with alcohol misuse who were not advised were in the mild-moderate alcohol misuse group. These data emphasize the importance of systematic alcohol screening and of standardizing the screening threshold for a performance measure of brief alcohol counseling.

A major strength of the SHEP survey for measuring performance of brief alcohol counseling is that it permits standardized assessment of both the denominator and the numerator. Moreover, use of surveys would focus clinicians and quality managers on implementing effective brief alcohol counseling that patients can recall rather than on increasing documentation of brief alcohol counseling per se. However, so far, only alcohol-related advice has been assessed, and no question about feedback has been tested (i.e., "In the past year, has your VA provider talked with you about how alcohol use can affect your health?"). Furthermore, stakeholders in the VA have been hesitant to use SHEP for a performance measure for brief alcohol counseling for two reasons. First, there is a lag-time before sites receive survey results

FIGURE 1. Patient reports of alcohol-related advice among VA outpatients who screened positive for alcohol misuse on surveys: the percent advised increased as AUDIT-C scores increased*

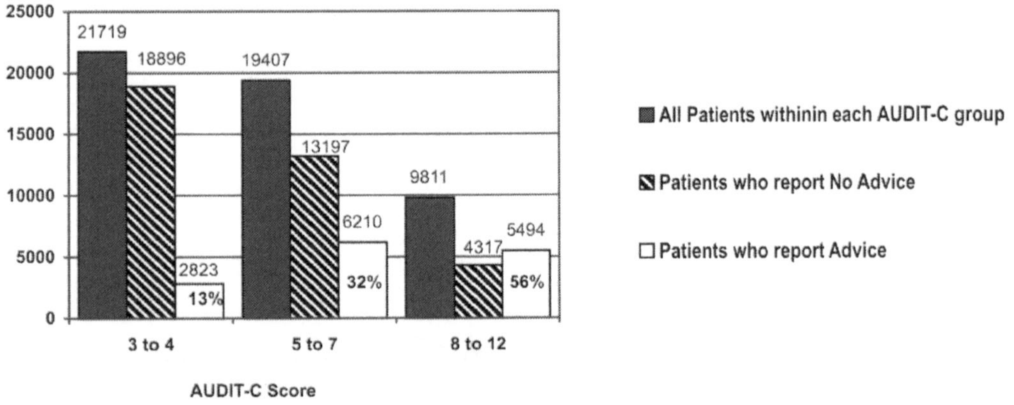

*Numbers based on VA SHEP survey in 2004. AUDIT-C scores of 3-4 suggest mild alcohol misuse (many patients who have these scores *report* drinking within recommended limits). AUDIT-C scores of 5-7 suggest mild/moderate alcohol misuse, most report drinking above recommended limits. AUDIT-C scores of 8-12 suggest severe alcohol misuse. Percentages on white bars indicate the percent of all patients in each AUDIT-C group who reported advice.

with no easy surrogate method for month-to-month monitoring for use in local quality improvement. Second, stakeholders have concerns about holding providers and managers accountable for counseling measured by patient report, which is susceptible to biases noted above.

Medical Record Documentation of Brief Alcohol Counseling. The VA contracts with an outside agency to conduct medical record reviews of a random sample of outpatients seen at each facility each month. This program is referred to as the External Peer Review Program (EPRP). Recently the VA OQP pilot-tested whether advice and feedback can be assessed with EPRP medical record reviews. The denominator of such a measure could be defined as patients who screened positive on the AUDIT-C based on medical record review. The numerator of the measure could reflect medical record documentation in the past year of: (1) advice to abstain or to drink within recommended limits and (2) feedback about the health risks of drinking (Figure 2). However, patients who reported drinking within recommended limits despite screening positive for alcohol misuse would only be required to have documentation of advice to maintain drinking below recommended limits. Determination of which patients had contraindications to drinking and should be advised to abstain could be left to provider discretion (Figure 2).

To determine whether documentation of these features of brief alcohol counseling could be routinely found by abstractors in the medical records of patients who screen positive for alcohol misuse, a 3-month pilot test of this measure was conducted without any interventions to increase brief alcohol counseling and without informing VA facilities and providers. Among 264 patients with documented severe alcohol misuse (AUDIT-C scores 8-12) whose charts

FIGURE 2. Elements of a pilot-tested measure of brief alcohol counseling based on EPRP* medical record review

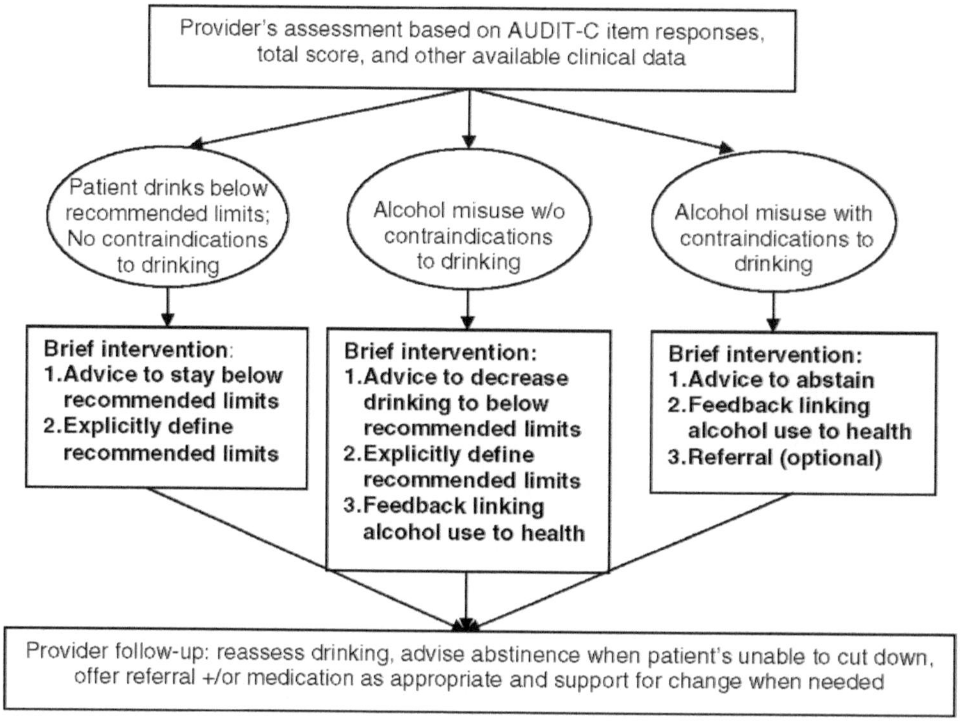

*EPRP=External Peer Review Program

were evaluated at least 30 days after alcohol screening, medical record review revealed the following components: advice to abstain (23.1%), advice to drink less (17.8%), personalized feedback linking alcohol use and health (18.9%), and general feedback on the association of alcohol use and health (19.3%). These data suggest that specific documentation of brief alcohol counseling can be abstracted from medical records.

Electronic Clinical Reminder to Prompt and Monitor Brief Alcohol Counseling. The VA's Computerized Patient Record System (CPRS) includes clinical reminders to prompt and monitor documented care. We developed and tested a CPRS clinical reminder for brief alcohol counseling, which is triggered electronically when patients screen positive on the AUDIT-C. The initial reminder was satisfied (e.g., turned off) if the provider documented alcohol-related advice alone, because formative evaluation suggested that requiring both advice and feedback might be a barrier to provider use of the reminder in the absence of any institutional incentive for brief alcohol counseling. Alcohol-related advice documented with the clinical reminder can be monitored by generating reports that indicate the proportion of patients with documented advice among those who screened positive for alcohol misuse.

We tested the reminder in an 8-site VA facility where providers were expected to use multiple clinical reminders. Results showed that it was acceptable to providers and was rapidly incorporated into care over a period of several months until leveling off at about two-thirds of screen-positive patients having brief alcohol advice documented with the reminder (Figure 3). This compares favorably to other brief alcohol counseling implementation efforts, which have resulted in rates of brief alcohol counseling from 13-60% (8). Figure 3 also demonstrates the sustainability of implementation and monitoring with clinical reminders. Furthermore, the proportion of patients who had documented brief alcohol counseling was about the

FIGURE 3. Electronic monitoring of use of a computerized clinical reminder (CR) to document brief alcohol-related advice at one 8-site VA facility: First 8 months after implementation of the clinical reminder*

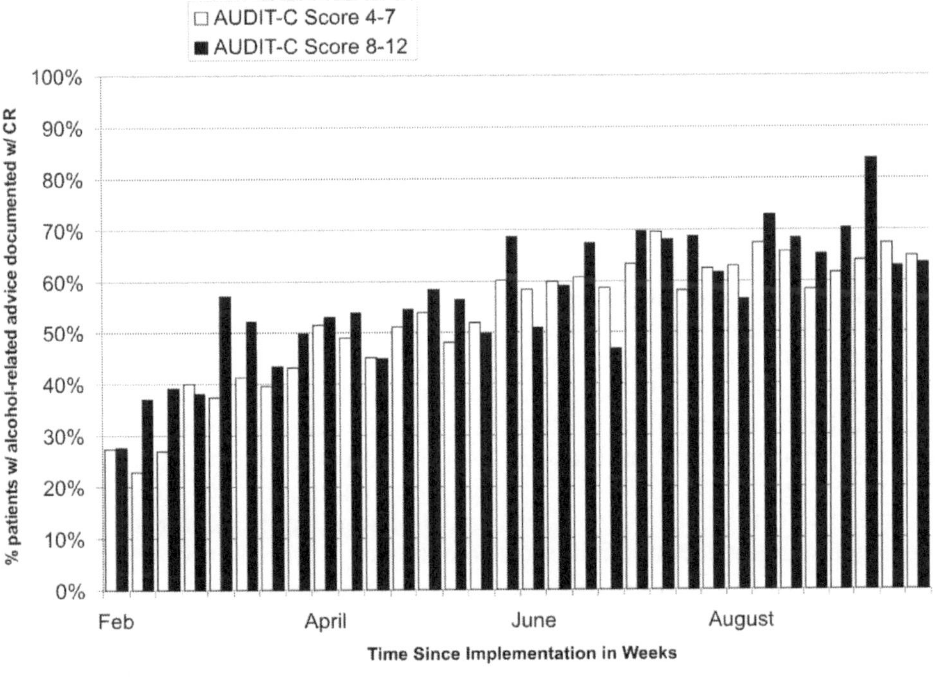

*Based on data from weekly clinical reminder reports from one VA facility in 2004. AUDIT-C scores 4-7 indicate mild/moderate alcohol misuse; AUDIT-C scores 8-12 indicate severe alcohol misuse.

same among patients with milder alcohol misuse as among those with severe alcohol misuse. Recently this clinical reminder has been modified to also require that patients receive either personalized or general feedback about the association between alcohol use and health, consistent with the above pilot-tested medical record review measure of brief alcohol counseling.

CONCLUSIONS AND RECOMMENDATIONS

Brief counseling for patients who misuse alcohol is one of the top 10 prevention priorities for the US (3). Such counseling decreases drinking, health care utilization and health care costs (4, 6). However, brief alcohol counseling has not been widely implemented (9). Development of a performance measure is essential for three reasons: to assess the proportion of patients with alcohol misuse who are offered brief alcohol counseling both within and across health care organizations, to promote implementation of high quality evidence-based brief alcohol counseling, and to evaluate whether targeted quality improvement efforts are effective (16, 74). However, there is currently no accepted performance measure of brief alcohol counseling.

For now, performance measures for brief alcohol counseling must be developed with incomplete evidence. There is no consensus on the single best alcohol screening test to identify patients with alcohol misuse or the required components of brief alcohol counseling. Further, the validity of provider and patient reports of brief alcohol counseling is not known. Therefore, this review of the issues and description of the VA experience are intended to stimulate and support further research efforts to identify and improve performance measures of brief alcohol counseling.

Administrative data often used for performance measurement cannot identify patients with alcohol misuse who should be offered brief alcohol counseling and cannot evaluate the quality of brief alcohol counseling provided. Moreover, use of administrative data could create unintended consequences: performance would appear better in settings that did not systematically screen for alcohol misuse, because patients with severe alcohol problems are most likely to be recognized and receive brief alcohol counseling in these settings. A performance measure based on administrative data would, therefore, risk penalizing health care systems for implementing recommendations for evidence-based alcohol screening (51, 75).

A specified alcohol screening questionnaire and screening threshold will be required to standardize the denominator of a performance measure of brief alcohol counseling. Otherwise, use of screening tests with varying sensitivity and specificity could lead to seemingly high rates of brief alcohol counseling in settings that excluded patients with less severe alcohol misuse from the denominator. However, the screening threshold for identifying the denominator of a performance measure for brief alcohol counseling may need to be less sensitive (slightly higher) than clinical screening thresholds to minimize the costs of false positive screens.

Research suggests that medical providers do not offer evidence-based brief alcohol counseling even when they discuss alcohol use with patients (58, 59). To encourage clinicians to provide evidence-based brief alcohol counseling, the numerator of a performance measure should not rely on non-specific provider documentation or patient reports that brief alcohol counseling occurred. Instead, a performance measure numerator should explicitly assess advice to drink below recommended limits or abstain and feedback linking alcohol use to health risks. These have been consistent components of brief alcohol interventions found efficacious in trials and could help distinguish evidence-based brief alcohol counseling from ineffective alcohol-related discussions.

A patient satisfaction survey like the CAHPS survey offers a feasible, readily available approach that can incorporate both standardized alcohol screening (2-3 questions) and assessment of key components of brief alcohol counseling (2 questions) across health care systems. Such an approach has the added advantage of easily permitting standardized measurement of alcohol misuse. Although surveys with adequate samples are expensive, the marginal cost of 4-5 questions is not high in systems with existing patient satisfaction surveys. If provider documentation is used to assess brief alcohol counseling, either by manual medical record review or electronic monitoring of medical record documentation, patient surveys could be used to validate provider documentation (67).

There are limits to what performance measurement alone can achieve. While performance measures of brief alcohol counseling will likely be required before brief alcohol counseling is implemented on a broad scale, they will not be sufficient. As shown by the VA experience in implementing routine alcohol screening with the AUDIT-C (9), a performance measure must be supplemented by system-wide education and continued quality improvement efforts. However, such quality improvement efforts for brief alcohol counseling can occur most effectively in the setting of high quality performance measurement.

In summary, an effective performance measure of brief alcohol counseling must specify an alcohol screening tool and threshold to identify a standardized denominator. An effective performance measure will also assess whether providers offer patients with alcohol misuse the two consistent components of efficacious brief alcohol counseling: advice about drinking limits and feedback on health risks of drinking. Mailed patient satisfaction surveys appear to provide the most readily available approach for collecting high quality data to compare performance of brief alcohol counseling across health care systems. More options are available for measuring performance of brief alcohol counseling within individual health care systems, especially those with electronic medical records.

REFERENCES

1. U.S. Preventive Services Task Force. Screening and behavioral counseling interventions in primary care to reduce alcohol misuse: Recommendation statement. Ann Intern Med. 2004;140:554-6.

2. VA Office of Quality and Performance. VA/DoD Clinical Practice Guidleline for the Management of Substance Use Disorders. http://www.oqp.med.va.gov/cpg/SUD/G/SUD%20PrimaryC%20Summary.pdf. 2001.

3. Maciosek MV, Coffield AB, Edwards NM, Flottemesch TJ, Goodman MJ, Solberg LI. Priorities among effective clinical preventive services results of a systematic review and analysis. Am J Prev Med. 2006; 31(1):52-61.

4. Fleming MF, Mundt MP, French MT, Manwell LB, Stauffacher EA, Barry KL. Benefit-cost analysis of brief physician advice with problem drinkers in primary care settings. Med Care. 2000;38(1):7-18.

5. Fleming MF, Barry KL, Manwell LB, Johnson K, London R. Brief physician advice for problem alcohol drinkers: a randomized controlled trial in community-based primary care practices. JAMA. 1997;277(13): 1039-45.

6. Fleming MF, Mundt MP, French MT, Manwell LB, Stauffacher EA, Barry KL. Brief physician advice for problem drinkers: long-term efficacy and benefit-cost analysis. Alcohol Clin Exp Res. 2002;26(1): 36-43.

7. Saitz R, Svikis D, D'Onofrio G, Kraemer KL, Perl H. Challenges applying alcohol brief intervention in diverse practice settings: populations, outcomes, and costs. Alcohol Clin Exp Res. 2006;30(2):332-8.

8. Nilsen P, Aalto M, Bendtsen P, Seppa K. Effectiveness of strategies to implement brief alcohol intervention in primary healthcare. A systematic review. Scand J Prim Health Care. 2006;24(1):5-15.

9. Bradley KA, Williams EC, Achtmeyer CE, Volpp B, Collins BJ, Kivlahan DR. Implementation of evidence-based alcohol screening in the Veterans Health Administration. Am J Manag Care. 2006;12(10): 597-610.

10. Institute of Medicine. Strengthening the Evidence Base and Quality Improvement Infrastructure. Improving the Quality of Health Care for Mental and Substance-Use Conditions. Washington, DC: The National Academies Press; 2006:140-209.

11. Blumenthal D. Part 1: Quality of care–what is it? N Engl J Med. 1996;335(12):891-4.

12. Brook RH, McGlynn EA, Cleary PD. Quality of health care. Part 2: measuring quality of care. N Engl J Med. 1996;335(13):966-70.

13. Asch SM, McGlynn EA, Hogan MA, et al. Comparison of quality of care for patients in the VHA and patients in a national sample. Ann Intern Med. 2004; 141(12):938-45.

14. McGlynn EA, Asch SM, Adams JL, et al. The quality of health care delivered to adults in the United States. N Engl J Med. 2003;348(26):2635-45.

15. Hermann RC, Palmer H, Leff S, et al. Achieving consensus across diverse stakeholders on quality measures for mental healthcare. Med Care. 2004;42(12): 1246-53.

16. Institute of Medicine. Improving the quality of mental health care for mental and substance-use conditions Washington DC: The National Academies Press; 2006. (Committee on Crossing the Quality Chasm: Adaptation to Mental Health and Addictive Disorders, ed. Quality Chasm Series).

17. Whitlock EP, Polen MR, Green CA, Orleans T, Klein J. Behavioral counseling interventions in primary care to reduce risky/harmful alcohol use by adults: A

summary of the evidence for the U.S. Preventive Services Task Force. Ann Intern Med. 2004;140:557-68.

18. Vinson DC, Mabe N, Leonard LL, et al. Alcohol and injury. Arch Fam Med. 1995;4:505-11.

19. Au DH, Kivlahan DR, Bryson CL, Blough D, Bradley KA. Alcohol screening scores and risk of hospitalization for GI conditions in men. Alcohol Clin Exp Res. 2007;31(3):443-51.

20. Moyer A, Finney JW, Swearingen CE, Vergun P. Brief interventions for alcohol problems: a meta-analytic review of controlled investigations in treatment-seeking and non-treatment-seeking populations. Addiction. 2002;97:279-92.

21. Ballesteros J, Duffy JC, Querejeta I, Arino J, Gonzalez-Pinto A. Efficacy of brief interventions for hazardous drinkers in primary care: Systematic review and meta-analyses. Alcohol Clin Exp Res. 2004;28(4): 608-18.

22. Wilk AI, Jensen NM, Havighurst TC. Meta-analysis of randomized control trials addressing brief interventions in heavy alcohol drinkers. J Gen Intern Med. 1997;12:274-283.

23. Walsh DC, Hingson RW, Merrigan DM, et al. The impact of a physician's warning on recovery after alcoholism treatment. JAMA. 1992;267:663-7.

24. Samet JH, Rollnick S, Barnes H. Beyond CAGE: a brief clinical approach after detection of substance abuse. Arch Intern Med. 1996;156:2287-2293.

25. Orford J, Hodgson R, Copello A, et al. The clients' perspective on change during treatment for an alcohol problem: qualitative analysis of follow-up interviews in the UK Alcohol Treatment Trial. Addiction. 2006;101(1):60-8.

26. Saitz R, Horton NJ, Sullivan LM, Moskowitz MA, Samet JH. Addressing alcohol problems in primary care: a cluster randomized, controlled trial of a systems intervention. The screening and intervention in primary care (SIP) study. Ann Intern Med. 2003;138(5):372-82.

27. Ockene JK, Adams A, Hurley TG, Wheeler EV, Hebert JR. Brief physician- and nurse practitioner-delivered counseling for high-risk drinkers. Arch Intern Med. 1999;159:2198-2205.

28. Babor TF, Higgins-Biddle JC, Dauser D, Burleson JA, Zarkin GA, Bray J. Brief interventions for at-risk drinking: patient outcomes and cost-effectiveness in managed care organizations. Alcohol Alcohol. 2006;41(6):624-31.

29. Burman ML, Kivlahan DR, Buchbinder MB, et al. Alcohol-related advice for VA primary care patients: who gets it, who gives it? J Stud Alc. 2004;65(5): 621-630.

30. Buchsbaum DG, Buchanan RG, Poses RM, Schnoll SH, Lawton MJ. Physician detection of drinking problems in patients attending a general medicine practice. J Gen Intern Med. 1992;7(5):517-521.

31. Volk RJ, Steinbauer JR, Cantor SB. Patient factors influencing variation in the use of preventive interventions for alcohol abuse by primary care physicians. J Stud Alcohol. 1996;57:203-209.

32. Kaner EF, Heather N, Brodie J, Lock CA, McAvoy BR. Patient and practitioner characteristics predict brief alcohol intervention in primary care. Br J Gen Pract. 2001;51(471):822-7.

33. Saitz R, Mulvey KP, Plough A, JH S. Physician unawareness of serious substance abuse. Am J Drug Alc Abuse. 1997;23:343-54.

34. Buchsbaum DG, Buchanan RG, Lawton MJ, Elswick RK Jr., Schnoll SH. A program of screening and prompting improves short-term physician counseling of dependent and nondependent harmful drinkers. Arch Intern Med. 1993;153(13):1573-77.

35. Wenrich MD, Paauw DS, Carline JD, Curtis JR, Ramsey PG. Do primary care physicians screen patients about alcohol intake using the CAGE questions? J Gen Intern Med. 1995;10:631-4.

36. Fleming MF. Strategies to increase alcohol screening in health care settings. Alcohol Res Health. 1997;21(4):340-7.

37. Kypri K, Langley JD, Saunders JB, Cashell-Smith ML. Assessment may conceal therapeutic benefit: findings from a randomized controlled trial for hazardous drinking. Addiction. 2007;102(1):62-70.

38. Coulton S, Drummond C, James D, et al. Opportunistic screening for alcohol use disorders in primary care: comparative study. BMJ. 2006;332(7540):511-7.

39. Taj N, Devera-Sales A, Vinson DC. Screening for problem drinking: does a single question work? J Fam Prac. 1998;46(4):328-35.

40. Williams R, Vinson DC. Validation of a single screening question for problem drinking. J Fam Pract. 2001;50(4):307-12.

41. Bradley KA, Bush K, Davis TD, et al. Two brief alcohol screening tests from the Alcohol Use Disorders Identification Test (AUDIT): validation in a female VA patient population. Arch Intern Med. 2003;163:821-39.

42. Bush KR, Kivlahan DR, McDonell MB, Fihn SD, Bradley KB. The AUDIT alcohol consumption questions (AUDIT-C): an effective brief screening test for problem drinking. Arch Intern Med. 1998;158: 1789-95.

43. Bradley KA, DeBenedetti AF, Volk RJ, Williams EC, Frank D, Kivlahan DR. AUDIT-C as a brief screen for alcohol misuse in primary care. Alcohol Clin Exp Res. 2007;31(7):1-10.

44. Dawson DA, Grant BF, Stinson FS. The AUDIT-C: screening for alcohol use disorders and risk drinking in the presence of other psychiatric disorders. Compr Psychiatry. 2005;46(6):405-16.

45. Dawson DA, Grant BF, Stinson FS, Zhou Y. Effectiveness of the derived Alcohol Use Disorders Identification Test (AUDIT-C) in screening for alcohol use disorders and risk drinking in the US general population. Alcohol Clin Exp Res. 2005;29(5):844-54.

46. Bradley KA, Kivlahan DR, Zhou XH, et al. Using alcohol screening results and treatment history to assess the severity of at-risk drinking in VA primary care patients. Alcohol Clin Exp Res. 2004;28(3):448-455.

47. Bradley KA, Maynard C, Kivlahan DR, McDonell MB, Fihn SD. The relationship between alcohol screening questionnaires and mortality among male VA outpatients. J Stud Alcohol. 2001;62:826-33.

48. Williams EC, Kivlahan DR, Saitz R, et al. Readiness to change in primary care patients who screened positive for alcohol misuse. Annals Fam Med. 2006; 4(3):213-20.

49. Walter LC, Davidowitz NP, Heineken PA, Covinsky KE. Pitfalls of converting practice guidelines into quality measures: lessons learned from a VA performance measure. JAMA. 2004;291(20):2466-70.

50. Grant BF, Stinson FS, Dawson DA, et al. Prevalence and co-occurrence of substance use disorders and independent mood and anxiety disorders: results from the National Epidemiologic Survey on Alcohol and Related Conditions. Arch Gen Psychiatry. 2004;61(8): 807-16.

51. U.S. Preventive Services Task Force. Guide to Clinical Preventive Services: Report of the U.S. Preventive Services Task Force, (DiGuiseppi C, Akins D, Woolf SH, eds.) Second Edition Baltimore: Williams and Wilkins; 1996.

52. Bertholet N, Daeppen JB, Wietlisbach V, Fleming M, Burnand B. Reduction of alcohol consumption by brief alcohol intervention in primary care: systematic review and meta-analysis. Arch Intern Med. 2005;1 65(9):986-95.

53. Bien TH, Miller WR, Tonigan S. Brief interventions for alcohol problems: a review. Addiction. 1993; 88:315-36.

54. Kahan M, Wilson L, Becker L. Effectiveness of physician-based interventions with problem drinkers. Can Med Assoc J. 1995;152(6):851-9.

55. Poikolainen K. Effectiveness of brief interventions to reduce alcohol intake in primary health care populations: a meta-analysis. Preventive Medicine. 1999;28:503-9.

56. Gentilello LM, Rivara FP, Donovan DM, et al. Alcohol intervention in a trauma center as a means of reducing the risk of injury recurrence. Ann Surg. 1999; 230(4):473-84.

57. WHO Brief Intervention Study Group. A cross-national trial of brief interventions with heavy drinkers. Am J Public Health. 1996;86(7):948-55.

58. Bradley KA, Epler A, Bush K, et al. Alcohol-related discussions during general medicine appointments of patients who screen positive for at-risk drinking. J Gen Intern Med. 2002;17(5):315-27.

59. McCormick KA, Cochran NE, Back AL, Merrill JO, Williams EC, Bradley KA. How primary care providers talk to patients about alcohol: A qualitative study. J Gen Intern Med. 2006;21:966-72.

60. Garnick DW, Lee MT, Chalk M, et al. Establishing the feasibility of performance measures for alcohol and other drugs. J Subst Abuse Treat. 2002;23(4):375-85.

61. Garnick DW, Horgan CM, Chalk M. Performance measures for alcohol and other drug services. Alcohol Research and Health. 2006;29(1):19-26.

62. Harris A, Humphreys K, Finney J. Veterans Affairs facility performance on Washington Circle indicators and casemix-adjusted effectiveness. JSAT. 2007. Mar 30; [Epub ahead of print]

63. Department of Health and Human Services. October Quarterly Update for 2006 Durable Medical Equipment, Prosthetics, Orthotics, and Supplies (DMEPOS) Fee Schedule. Centers for Medicare and Medicaid Services. 2006:http://www.cms.hhs.gov/transmittals/downloads/R1037CP.pdf.

64. Saitz R. Clinical practice. Unhealthy alcohol use. N Engl J Med. 2005;352(6):596-607.

65. NCQA. HEDIS 2007 Specifications for Survey Measures. Vol. 3 http://www.ncqa.org/communications/publications/hedispub.htm#HED3; 2007.

66. Tisnado DM, Adams JL, Liu H, et al. What is the concordance between the medical record and patient self-report as data sources for ambulatory care? Med Care. 2006;44(2):132-40.

67. Hawkins E, Kivlahan D, Williams E, Wright S, Craig T, Bradley K. Examining quality issue in alcohol misuse screening. Substance Abuse. 2007; 28(3):53-65.

68. Perlin JB, Kolodner RM, Roswell RH. The Veterans Health Administration: quality, value, accountability, and information as transforming strategies for patient-centered care. Am J Manag Care. 2004;10(11 Pt 2):828-36.

69. Stange KC, Zyznaski SJ, Smith TF, et al. How valid are medical records and patient questionnaires for physician profiling and health services research? Med Care. 1998;36(6):851-67.

70. Dexter PR, Perkins S, Overhage JM, Maharry K, Kohler RB, McDonald CJ. A computerized reminder system to increase the use of preventive care for hospitalized patients. N Engl J Med. 2001;345(13):965-70.

71. Weiner M, Callahan CM, Tierney WM, et al. Using information technology to improve the health care of older adults. Ann Intern Med. 2003;139(5 Pt 2):430-6.

72. Yarnall KSH, Pollak KI, Ostbye T, Krause KM, Micchener JL. Primary care: Is there enough time for prevention? Am J Public Health. 2003;93(4):635-41.

73. Tanne JH. UK fares well in survey of primary care, but US doesn't. BMJ. 2006;333(7576):985.

74. Institute of Medicine. Achieving a National System for Performance Measurement and Reporting. Performance Measurement: Accelerating Improvement. Washington, DC: The National Academies Press; 2006: 63-82.

75. U.S. Department of Health and Human Services, Public Health Service, National Institutes of Health, National Institute on Alcohol Abuse and Alcoholism. The Physicians' Guide to Helping Patients with Alcohol Problems NIH; 1995.

doi:10.1300/J465v28n04_05

Index

Page numbers followed by a *t* or *f* indicate tables or figures.